Maurice Mességué's
Way to Natural
Health and Beauty

By the same author
Of Men and Plants

Maurice Mességué's
Way to Natural Health and Beauty

MAURICE MESSEGUE

Translated from the French by

CLARA WINSTON

Macmillan Publishing Co., Inc.

NEW YORK

Macmillan Publishing Co., Inc.
866 Third Avenue, New York,
N.Y. 10022

Library of Congress Cataloging in Publication Data

Mességué, Maurice.
    Maurice Mességué's way to natural health and beauty.

    Translation of C'est la nature qui à raison.
    1. Nutrition. 2. Hygiene. 3. Cookery, French.
I. Title. II. Title: Way to natural health and
beauty. [DNLM: 1. Diet. 2. Hygiene. 3. Nutrition.
QT235 M584c 1974]
RS164.M39313   613.2   74-8944
ISBN 0-02-584370-2

This book was originally
published in France under the title
C'est la nature qui à raison.

First Printing 1974
Printed in the United States of America

To E.A.
With all my gratitude

Contents

1. Pollution: The Evil Spell   1

2. Man and Nature: A Time of Rediscovery   13

3. Cultivate Your Garden   33
Garlic. Onion. Cabbage. Carrot. Celery. Watercress. Lettuce. Cucumber. Artichoke. Tomato. Spinach. Chicory. Dandelion. Radish. Fennel. Asparagus. Turnip and Rutabaga. Rhubarb. Strawberry and Raspberry. Currant and Gooseberry. Blackberry. Blueberry. Apple. Cherry. Peach, Apricot and Pear. Plum. Grape.

4. The Secrets of Herbs   74
Parsley and Chervil. Thyme. Rosemary. Sage. Savory. Bay Leaf. Basil. Tarragon, Marjoram. Mint. Nettles. Celandine. Pimpernel. Lavender. Couch Grass. Ivy. Mallow. Poppy. Shepherd's Purse. Rose. Violet. Nasturtium. Hawthorn. Borage. Yarrow. Cowparsnip. Corn Silk.

5. Sickness: An Alarm Signal   119
The Liver. The Stomach. The Intestines. The Kidneys and Bladder. Rheumatism. The Respiratory Tract. Allergies. Nervous Complaints. Sexual Problems. The Heart and the Circulatory System.

6. Beauty: A Promise of Happiness   154
Cellulite. The Skin. The Face. The Eyes. The Teeth and Mouth. The Hair.

7. **Tell Me What You Eat**   177
*Meats. Seafood. Bread and Cereals. Dairy Products.
Sweets. Beverages.*

8. **A Sheaf of Favorite Recipes**   194
Soups: *Garlic Soup. Aïgo Bouïdo. Creamed Onion Soup.
Creamed Garlic Soup. Soupe de Vie. Soupe au Farci.
Sour-Milk Soup. Cherry Soup. Queen Margot's
Potage. Sunday Night Soup. Chicory Potage. "Little
Cousin" or Mallow Soup. Purslane Soup. Tarragon
Soup. Pea-pod Soup. Nettle Soup. Radish-top Soup.
A Meatless Pot-au-feu. Cold Sorrel Soup. Gazpacho.
Vegetable Juice.*
Main Dishes: *Boiled Chicken, Henri IV Style. Galimfrey.
Rabbit with Prunes. Stuffed Poultry with Prunes.
Chicken with Capon. Pot Roast, Polish Style. Herb
Omelette. Velvet Eggs. Onion Tart. Chicken with
Onions. Stuffed Breast of Veal. Carbonade. Gascon-
nade. Roast Pork with Herbs. Marinated Pork Roast.
Salmagundi.*
Sauces: *Mint Sauce. Sage Sauce. Herb Sauce for Fish.
Green Sauce. Mixed Herb Sauce. Poor Man's Sauce.
Garlic Butter. Currant Sauce. Rosehip Sauce. Holy
Water Sauce. Pimpernel Sauce.*
Vegetables: *Stuffed Cabbage. Stuffed Cabbage with
Chestnuts. Eggplant Caviar. Cabbage with Milk.
Cabbage with Onions. Red Cabbage with Apples.
Puréed Onions. Onions in the Embers. Eggplant,
Squash or Tomatoes in the Embers. Beans with
Savory. Hops à la Vinaigrette. Lettuce au gratin.
Stuffed Lettuce. Purslane au gratin. Fresh Peas with
Mint. Beet Greens. Coconut and Vegetable Pudding.
Rhubarb Blossom au gratin. Dandelion Salad with
Croutons. Grapefruit Salad Dressing. Red Cabbage
Salad, Heated. Marinated Cucumbers. American
Salad Bowl and Dip.*
Desserts: *Clafouti. Candied Carrots. Chestnuts with
Fennel. Raisiné. A Simpler Raisiné. Cider Jam. Elder-
berry Jam. Carrot Jam. Honey Jam. Acacia Flower*

Fritters. Rose Custard. Orange Blossom Custard. Violet Paste. Jasmine Paste. Candied Orange Blossoms.

Beverages: *Gentian Wine. Marjoram Milk. Eggnog. Mulled Wine. Rose Honey. Blueberry Syrup. Orange Blossom* Ratafia. *Rose* Ratafia. *Hippocras. Ambrosia. Bachelor's Liqueur.*

9. **A Way of Life After My Heart** 230

Index 245

1. Pollution: The Evil Spell

I was born in a tiny village called Gavarret in the Gers in France. Some people say I am always going on about my childhood and my village, but I find it necessary to go far back to reach the source of personal knowledge. At any rate, at Gavarret there were more animals than people, I do not mean only farm animals but also a multitude of small creatures of every sort which gave the village the character of Noah's Ark teeming with its passengers. Man and beasts lived together in relative harmony, despite certain natural differences of interest. I could not, for instance, take my nap in the shade of a hedge on a summer's day because of the commotion of the birds nesting in the thicket. When I went herb-gathering, I would be quite annoyed at the number of rabbit holes everywhere, for the rabbits were interested in many of the same herbs as I was.

Nowadays, I am shocked when I return to these places of which I have such happy memories. There are no rabbit holes in the fields or birds in the hedges. Many other kinds of animals have also disappeared—specialists have listed 120 species of mammals and 250 species of birds that have disappeared from the face of the earth in the past few decades. Noah's Ark is becoming empty and man finds himself more and more alone.

What has happened? What has shattered this natural idyll? What evil spell has blasted the good earth that gave shelter to so many forms of life? In the old days the country people believed in evil spells and in the mischief done by witches. Nowadays in this age of reason and science we are told that evil spells and witches are products of man's imagination and are not to be feared. But in fact we are afraid, and with good cause, when confronted with the mysterious bane that has fallen upon the things of nature. By now we are all aware that the terrible poisoning of earth, air and water that we call Pollution must be checked, and as soon as possible. We cannot let this process take its course, for the future of the globe itself is in danger. Surely, here is a threat more dire and far-reaching than any a band of witches could have posed. In the Middle Ages a community stricken by evils it could not understand would hold a public hearing, charge some of its womenfolk with witchcraft and in due course burn the "offenders" in the public square. But rituals such as these do not banish the evil of pollution.

Still and all, the need to take defensive action is greater than ever, so I decided to convoke a meeting in the good town of Fleurance, of which I have the honor to be mayor. This is how the National Conference for the Defense of Nature met in Fleurance on June 27, 1971. I assembled a panel of experts—doctors, biologists, biochemists, agronomists. Also invited were a number of prominent jurists and public figures who could be helpful in putting the findings of the conference into practical form. And since the questions to be discussed were of the utmost concern to all and sundry, I also invited the general public. The result was that we had some fifteen hundred persons there.

In view of the large attendance and in keeping with the spirit of the occasion, the meeting was held out of doors in the town's market square. The setting was highly appropriate, for overlooking our square is a thirteenth-century fortress which, in the days when it was built, would have given shelter to the entire population of the town and surrounding countryside in case of attack. And are we not nowadays under attack, faced by a threat more cunning and more destructive than any of the past? I was very pleased to see that a large proportion of the townspeople had come to the meeting, and filled the square to capacity, ready to take arms against the common enemy.

I had made a point of massing flowers everywhere—around the handsome fountain of the market square, around the stone water basins on the side streets and on the balconies of the Hôtel de Ville. My councilmen were rather dubious. "Isn't this going a bit too far, Your Honor? So many flowers for a town the size of ours—think of the cost!" But I have always set great store by flowers, and how much more so for an occasion like this one, when we were taking our stand against the forces that menace the flowering earth. I felt very strongly that this was no time to stint on tubs of geraniums and pots of carnations.

In the Middle Ages people tried to protect themselves from the miasmas of the plague by breathing the clean fragrance of mint and other pungent herbs. In Arab lands mint is still strewn in the marketplace as a public health measure. The town of Fleurance experienced a siege of plague in the seventeenth century, and the story of how mint was used as a disinfectant still lives in the popular mind. So I knew that on this score I would have popular support for my lavish use of flowers.

People sometimes criticize me for building my theories on small details of this kind. I must admit that I do place considerable emphasis on details, for I am a simple man for whom the tree is a more vivid presence than the forest, who feels worse about the single bird I find dead in the fields than about the statistics presented by experts on species decimated by pollution. To me, the pot of flowers set out on the balcony of a simple house in Fleurance seemed every bit as significant as the resolutions passed by our dignified assembly. Before the meeting started, I went around the town counting the flowerpots, and I knew that the town was with me. As far as Fleurance was concerned, the death sentence had been passed against Pollution.

Why, then, all the to-do about the conference, since I knew already what the verdict would be? Because I need the opinions of experts to confirm my own conviction. People are always asking me for proofs of my theories. But I am sadly lacking in such proofs. I know certain things by instinct, but I cannot prove them. That is how I perform my cures and that is how I conduct my life—purely by instinct.

Nevertheless, the panel of experts were at no loss for data and proof, statistics and extrapolations, and what they had to say that day in Fleurance should have made the whole world tremble. They conjured up scenes out of the Apocalypse—rivers poisoned, lands turned to desert, forests withered, animals annihilated and starving human beings crippled by all manner of diseases wandering through a barren landscape whose very atmosphere had turned to toxic gases.

I will not repeat all they said—enough articles and books have been published so that everyone should be informed on the problem. But I was greatly interested in what various local people at the conference had to say about their own experiences with pollution. Twenty years ago, when I began to talk about these dangers, I felt like a voice crying in the wilderness. Today so many farmers and so many experts testify to the same facts that it takes no special boldness to cry: We must put an end to pollution before it puts an end to us! If we go on the way we have been going, we are finished.

I, too, have had certain experiences that underline the danger we are in. Recently two of my small flock of hens, perfectly healthy birds that had been scratching happily in their little poultry yard, d'ed suddenly. I called in the veterinarian. "Your hens have been eating grain treated against weevils," he told me. I immediately destroyed two sacks of grain I had just bought, for I was not going to risk losing my other hens, or what was more serious, worrying about my children's getting sick from the eggs of these hens.

My two dead hens were victims of the reckless use of insecticides. To be sure, weevils are a serious menace to agriculture, along with innumerable other bugs and worms. But the measures taken against such insects have become a plague in themselves. I know certain housewives who run for their insect bombs whenever they see a single spider or fly inside their homes. Then they come to me for advice because their children have eczema, their husbands asthma and they themselves are prey to various allergies. They see no connection between these ailments and their war against insects. But I do.

To be sure, few of us today are troubled by head lice, fleas in our mattresses or the good old bedbugs for which brothels were famous (brothels themselves have gone out of style). By and large we live hygienically and pride ourselves on our clean skins. But our tissues and organs are saturated with all kinds of dangerous substances that we have absorbed without being aware of it. Fortunately for us, these enter our systems in minute amounts. However, every so often an accident occurs that points up the risk we are constantly running. Here is something that happened to some friends of mine, city people who rented a country place for the summer, not far from Fleurance.

My friends were thrilled to find a tree on their property bowed down with beautiful blue plums. As the fruit ripened in the rich sunlight, they conceived the idea of making some preserves to take back to the city as a souvenir of their country stay. Before bottling the preserves, they could not resist the temptation to sample some. One hour later the entire family had to be rushed to the hospital at Toulouse with all the symptoms of poisoning. It was later discovered that the owner of the country house had sprayed his plum tree just before my friends rented the place, and had forgotten to mention the matter to his tenants. Fortunately, they survived this mishap, but one can easily imagine how it could have been fatal.

I do not know too much about chemistry and could not easily find my way among the staggering array of sprays and dusts available to the general public. However, when I look over the labels on the shelf of the local hardware store, I am struck by the large number that contain some form or other of arsenic. Certain labels, while listing more innocuous substances, will nevertheless carry warnings of this sort:

> Do not eat, drink or smoke while applying this product.
> Wear protective clothing, rubber gloves and a cap with visor.
> Care should be taken not to inhale any of the spray during application.
> Wash exposed skin thoroughly with soap and water after working with this product.
> In case of discomfort, call a doctor.
> Do not discard any leftover solution into streams.
> Keep out of reach of children and livestock.
> All vessels and containers should be thoroughly rinsed after use.
> Destroy all empty cartons.
> Under certain conditions, there is a danger that herbicidal hormones in this product may affect nearby crops. Every precaution should be taken to prevent drift of this product. Use only on windless days, and when the temperature does not exceed 95 degrees.
> Do not store near grain or other foodstuffs.
> Inflammable.
> Do not freeze.

Most of the labels are decorated with an expressive death's head and carry a line to the effect that the manufacturer declines all responsibility for accidents resulting from use of the product. There is also apt to be a fifteen-day clause—the warning to the grower that the spraying program must be discontinued fifteen days before harvest time. It is hard to understand why something that is a dangerous poison on the fourteenth day may be considered harmless on the sixteenth day. We may also wonder what happens when the grower loses count, or when there is some upset in his harvesting plan. For agriculture does not lend itself to such exactitude. Nor is there any way to check on how carefully such warnings are followed.

All in all, the possibility of poisoning from chemical sprays and dusts is not inconsiderable. Farmers themselves, particularly fruit growers, are exposed to a host of diseases that can all be traced to the same cause—the chemicals with which they have to work. There have been many scientific investigations of this subject, and most farmers are well aware of the dangers. But the consumer must also be made aware of this problem.

These chemical products fall into three categories—fungicides, herbicides and insecticides. On the face of it, these represent a valuable arsenal against the endless pests the farmer has to deal with. But here too certain questions have arisen, which I can best illustrate by an anecdote.

My cousin, Michel Descamps, still lives in my native village of Gavarret and farms his family property. He often talks to me about his troubles.

"Maurice," he told me a few years ago, "I really don't know what to do. Ever since I took over the farm I have been spraying my vines against the grape worm. Well, the worms seem to have been wiped out but the red spiders have come in something fierce and they do a lot more damage than the worms ever did."

"Shouldn't you use another type of spray?"

"But there is no spray against red spiders. They resist everything."

Each spring I asked my cousin how he was getting on with his red spider problem. About two years ago Michel was becoming desperate.

"You know, Maurice, I have just about had enough. I am going to try an experiment. I am going to cut down on my spraying program and see what happens."

I asked him to keep me informed on how things were going. Now, two years later, Michel is much more cheerful. The spiders have disappeared from his vines. The grape worm is back, but not in such numbers as to be a problem. Just what happened? I myself would say that the natural balance had been righted. Entomologists would explain it somewhat differently. They would point out that there were two species of insects involved here, one of which preyed upon the other. When one species was eliminated by chemical sprays, the other, which no longer had any natural enemies, increased unchecked. They would also point out that many species of insects are capable of developing chemical-resistant strains. The same is true of many viruses, which have rapidly evolved new forms resistant to antibiotics. Scientists call this the "theory of adaptive radiation." When I speak of the balance of nature, I suppose I am referring to the same thing.

But to get back to my cousin Michel. Like all farmers, he has many problems. Yet now that he had his vines under control, I was surprised to see him looking gloomy. "What is it, Michel?" I asked him. "Is the baby sick or something?"

"No, Maurice," he answered. "It is my fields that are sick. I've been trying to doctor them, but the more medicines I give them, the worse they get."

"In what way?" I asked.

"It is mostly my wheat fields," he said. "They used to be full of poppies and cornflowers and thistles. Pretty to look at, but no way to grow wheat. So I tried some of this new herbicide that you spread at planting time. The first year it worked fine. The second year there were no poppies and cornflowers and thistles but there was plenty of foxtail and wild oat. And once that wild oat comes in, it can ruin a whole field of wheat."

"So you went to your farm dealer and asked for something to use on foxtail and wild oat."

"Yes, that's just what I asked for. He sold me some other stuff, but it seems there isn't anything you can do about foxtail and wild oat. So I've been spreading those fields with more and more chemicals every year and the weeds come in worse and worse."

Michel, like other farmers, has been caught in a vicious cycle. Every year vaster quantities of chemicals are used in agriculture.

The same fields are being asked to support greater yields of the same crops. And the soil grows tired, as we ourselves feel tired after a long illness in which we have been heavily dosed with medicines.

We know beyond question that if chemical fertilizers were suddenly withheld from our fields, their yield would be far lower than it was in the days before we came to depend upon such fertilizers. Productive though the soil may seem at present, it is basically exhausted because it is never allowed to rest. We have poured on the fertilizer and taken pride in the resultant bumper crops. But nothing has been done to restore the original fertility of the soil.

Meanwhile, the blights and weeds and insect pests multiply, for the plants have lost their innate sturdiness and the depleted soil is no longer a source of vitality but an artificial medium for holding chemicals. Everything has been sacrificed to productivity, and now that productivity is threatened. So the farmer has no choice but to shower his crops with chemicals. Because these products are costly, he has to realize a greater return on his land. In seeming to lower his risk, the farmer has in fact greatly increased his risk.

To complicate his life further, the farmer has to become something of an expert in a field in which he does not easily feel at home. He must study agricultural textbooks and mull over the difficult language of folders, for every product has to be handled differently and mistakes can cost him dearly. Certain herbicides, for example, have an active life of six months, others of a year or more. Besides, their effect on different crops is by no means uniform. A field planted to corn and treated with a herbicide designed to keep down weeds and eliminate the need for cultivation will have to lie fallow for two years before it can be planted to any other grain, for the herbicide in question is very longlasting and will kill any grasses. We should realize that all grains (with the exception of corn) are essentially grasses. Thus the question of succession plantings becomes a highly complicated one and the old principle of rotating crops, for so long one of the basic laws of agriculture, is apt to go by the board.

When I was a boy I knew all the springs and brooks around Gavarret and used to love to drink from them, cupping the crystal-clear water in my palms. Nowadays the farmers put up barbed wire around these same springs and brooks to keep their sheep from getting poisoned. For the chemicals used in agriculture find their way into all the local water sources and have by now accumulated to a dangerous extent.

But we are all aware that the world's water is no longer healthful and cleansing. The rivers in which we used to swim are contaminated by industrial waste and raw sewage. Vast oil slicks cover the ocean and black tides wash up on our beaches. Even the air we breathe is toxic, from the fumes of cars and industrial plants. We do not know what to do with the waste products of our civilization. And here once again human carelessness compounds the evil. The farmer tosses the empty carton of insecticide into a brook. The small community allows its sewers to empty into the nearest stream. The factory discharges its wastes into a river. In every case everyone does what is easiest and lets others reap the consequences. But the others are all of us who inhabit this once-fair earth.

I am not good at remembering large figures. But I have not forgotten one statistic mentioned to me by a good friend of mine, Pierre Pasquini, back in 1964 when he was vice president of the French National Assembly. The first legislation to protect the environment had just been passed and a study had been made to determine the amount of waste disgorged annually into the rivers of France.

"Maurice," my friend asked, "have you any idea of the quantities involved?"

I had to admit that I hadn't.

"Well, it comes to about six million tons, or the contents of ten thousand freight cars."

Ever since then I have been haunted by the image of those ten thousand freight cars vomiting their filth into our rivers, the beautiful rivers of France whose course we used to trace on the map in school and whose names alone were full of poetry.

Recently Pasquini, who is a lawyer as well as a fervent conservationist, told me about a case he had just undertaken on the basis of the new laws. "This is a very sad business," he said. "The victim is a small river in Haute Provence, the Isole. One day some anglers reported that the stream was full of dead trout. Investigations were made and eventually it was discovered that several miles upstream a few men had been rinsing snail shells in chlorine and dumping the water back into the stream. Again a whole river poisoned by human carelessness! Well, now at least we have a few laws on the books which make that sort of thing a punishable offense."

I was talking to another friend who lives near Grasse, the small town in the south of France where the perfume industry is largely centered. "You're a lucky fellow," I said, "to be living surrounded by fields of flowers."

"Not so lucky at all," he answered. "Didn't you know that the pollution level at Grasse is one of the worst in the country? The discharges of the perfume plants are extremely high in chemicals, and all our local rivers have been contaminated. There have also been bad effects on people and animal life, so that our area has become very pollution-conscious."

I could hardly believe my ears, for Grasse had always seemed to me the most idyllic place to live, surrounded by jasmine and roses. And now the roses themselves had become a bane. How could roses be harmful? They were so lovely to look at, their petals so silken, their fragrance so heavenly. I have always made a cult of roses and can never have enough of them around me. Now even flowers can be the agent of this new plague called Pollution, which conceals itself in so many forms.

I was talking to some of the farmers at the cattle fair in Fleurance. I complimented them on the appearance of their cows—they did indeed seem magnificent animals. But the farmers themselves took a more skeptical line toward their prized livestock. "Our animals are not what they used to be, Your Honor," they told me. "They used to be strong and tough. Today you have to watch over them constantly. They get sick from every little thing, and you are always calling in the veterinary. If one of these days we had a gasoline shortage in France and had to give up our tractors, there wouldn't be a single pair of oxen in the whole country fit to drag a plow."

One of the most dangerous aspects of modern agriculture is the use of antibiotics on farm animals. The purpose of this is twofold—to protect the animals against disease and to speed up their growth. To these ends the grain companies have spiked most feed mixtures with chemical substances. To be sure, the farmer is pleased that it takes less time to ready a hog for market and that his calves weigh in at higher levels than they used to. But the animals have become prone to many organic disturbances that were unknown in the past. Some years ago there was a general scare over the use of sex hormones in poultry production—consumers were rightly alarmed over the effects of estrogen on their own constitutions. In response to the public outcry a law was passed in 1965 in France banning the use of estrogen in animal feeds. Nevertheless, the law is often flouted, and every year government inspection turns up some fifteen thousand calves that have been given hormone injections. It would appear that with the increase of artificial means to fatten animals and raise the farmer's profit, there has been a corresponding increase in fraud.

Such abuse of antibiotics has a number of sinister effects on human health. For one thing, people develop allergies toward many kinds of food. But there is an even more serious consequence. When people become saturated with certain antibiotics, these lose their efficacy in emergencies. It is useless for a doctor to prescribe a certain medicine for a disease when the patient has been taking it more or less as his daily fare. But most dangerous of all is the threat of cancer. Every day scientists discover more carcinogenic substances to which we are all exposed. By now we are generally aware of the role played by cigarettes and industrial fumes in the genesis of cancer, but the chemical substances in our food, the traces of fertilizers and insecticides that build up in our tissues, can also create precancerous conditions. The list of dangerous additives is forever mounting—the coloring matter used in baking and candy-making, the artificial flavorings used in frozen desserts, the ripening agents sprayed on fruit, the alkalines and acids used in carbonated beverages and the host of preservatives the food industry adds to all its products. Even wine, once the pure juice of the grape and a source of vitality to our forbears, has become a laboratory creation treated with everything under the sun. A bottle of white wine sometimes contains more sulphur than a book of matches. Sulphur, apparently, helps wine keep. Whether it helps us keep is another question.

When we read a list of the chemicals which may legally be added to wine, we have a right to be horrified. That the law limits the quantities is a small consolation.

The time has come to demand better laws. We must speak out against this excessive processing of our food and drink. We must also protest against all those things done in the name of progress that are rapidly leading to the ruination of nature. We must each use what weapons we have—our power as consumers and voters, our influence on our neighbors, our moral force and our concern for the future of our children. Every blow in this cause has an impact, whether we organize a major campaign or spearhead a small boycott. We must fight pollution on every front and in every form. We must drive it out of our country and encourage our neighbors to do the same. Only a vigilant Interpol will protect the planet from this enemy, which mocks at borders and steals across continents and oceans in winds and tides.

We must not slacken our efforts until we have attained total victory.

2. Man and Nature: A Time of Rediscovery

It is easy to lament our present impasse but more important to look for a way out of it. The tendency nowadays is to accept the darkest prediction as final: "What's the use of struggling? Pollution is here to stay. It is the curse of our time and there's nothing we can do about it."

But man has always struggled when his survival was at stake. Fear has always been the greatest spur to action. It sharpens the brains of the most careless-minded, and in time of war gives rise to countless acts of heroism. The comparison with wartime is appropriate, for pollution is our common enemy and its ravages are greater even than those of war. But the awareness of danger is the beginning of wisdom. Someone who has seen an auto accident will drive more carefully, and someone who has seen his chickens poisoned by chemically-treated grain will be more concerned about the purity of the food he gives his children.

Today we believe in frankness. Doctors are inclined to give their patients a truthful picture of their condition so that they can come to terms with the facts, make the necessary decisions and do what is best for their families. And sometimes in meeting this challenge, the patient draws upon an inner force that enables him to reverse the tide and bit by bit beat back the illness.

This is how we must deal with pollution. We must first assess the full extent of the danger. To be sure, the major actions will have to be taken by governments. But public opinion is of the utmost importance, for the impetus to start the movement and sustain it must come from the people as a whole. In France we have now established a Ministry of Nature, which has wide powers. The great question is where to start, for there is so much to be done, so much information to gather, so many regulations to draw up.

Slow as France has been to move in this realm, she has now awakened to the urgency of the problem. This has not yet happened on the international scene. We might have expected the United Nations to take the leadership in a worldwide campaign for the defense of the environment, but instead that body has come out for an enormous increase in the use of fertilizers and insecticides in the underdeveloped countries. True, the most pressing need in those parts of the world is to control insect-borne diseases and raise agricultural production. Therefore, there is less concern with obtaining pure and healthful food than with overcoming starvation. I can well understand this point of view. In traveling through some of the poorer countries, I have been stricken at the sight of native children, so thin, with such big eyes in pinched little faces. At such times I hardly dare think of the array of foodstuffs we have at home. It seems quite impossible to say: "The problem is not quantity but quality." Or: "Our chief concern must be the protection of the environment." No, looking at these children one feels that all the peoples of the world must pitch in and raise the largest crops they can, so that the rich lands can give to the poor lands.

Alas, that is not how our present system operates. Too often I have seen truckloads of cauliflowers, tomatoes or peaches dumped by the wayside by angry farmers unable to sell their too bountiful harvest. When I see such a sight, I remember what parents used to say to children who would crumble up their bread at table: "Think of the starving children of India." That used to be a standard household phrase.

The sad fact is that those who have too much cannot take care of those who have too little. Not only distance, but all kinds of political, economic and commercial problems separate the starving Biafran child from the beautiful peaches crushed by the roadside in France. But even so, this matter must weigh on our consciences, we cannot thrust it from our minds. It can serve as a good corrective to whatever conceit we may feel at living in a rich country or whatever illusions we may have as to how philanthropic we are.

Neither should this problem prevent us from viewing our own plight realistically. There is overwhelming evidence that in our march toward progress we have taken the wrong road. We must now retrace our way and head in a different direction. Up to this time the sole objective has been quantity. From now on it must be quality *plus* quantity. To concentrate exclusively on quality would be another mistake, for we have not yet reached the point where the basic needs of mankind are being adequately met—that is still far in the future. But we must work toward that goal without further damage to the balance of nature. Once we are fully committed to this task, we must trust that our scientists will solve these problems of production and environmental protection, and that our governments will find the way to implement the solutions. After all, in its long history mankind has solved far more difficult problems.

It seems a pity that the best scientific talent of our time should be squandered on superfluous projects like the conquest of space when there are so many pressing problems on our own planet. It is more important to attain good health than to reach the moon. I do not mean only one's own health and that enjoyed by the fortunate members of society, but the health of all human beings, the poor in our midst and the countless inhabitants of the Third World who are still condemned to live in wretchedness. We must want to see the animals thriving, too, both the creatures of the wild and of the barnyard, who have for so long been mankind's friends. We ought to think also of the birds and butterflies and flowers that bring so much beauty into our lives. Perhaps society as a whole should set up priorities. I suggest that we put health first and foremost and assign a lower priority to mere technical feats. I have already mentioned moon flights as an example of an unnecessary and prodigiously costly venture. The list of what society can do without might also include fancier autos (to go where in an increasingly blighted world?), endless household gadgets (which add nothing to our domestic happiness) and the countless trashy novelties that crowd the stores (whose profits profit us not at all).

Once we have agreed on the goals of health and happiness—and surely we can all fundamentally agree on these—let us see how our ideal can be attained. Possible action ranges all the way from measures taken on an international scale to efforts we can make as individuals. The latter is where I can offer some suggestions. In my practice as a healer I have found that a profound connection exists between human well-being and the properties of plants. I am convinced that similar connections and affinities prevail between all forms of life. We must trust nature more, discover her laws and try to live in conformity with them. This calls for a good deal of research and experiment along lines I will describe later. But first let me tell you of an experiment I recently carried out in my own town of Fleurance.

For me, the function of mayor does not consist of closeting myself in my office and signing papers all day. To be sure, the Fleurance town hall is a handsome old building which is a joy to spend time in. I especially appreciate it during our Gascon summers when the thick stone walls keep it cool. The view from the town hall balcony is especially fine and I love to look down at the market square lined with dignified eighteenth-century houses. But I am not the sort of official who makes public appearances on the balcony. I am much more apt to be down in the square, or strolling about the streets and having a word with the townspeople. I want to find out whether the citizens of Fleurance are happy and whether there is anything I as mayor can do to improve the life of the town.

Each man has his individual joys and sorrows, but when one speaks to many, one begins to have a sense of the common lot. The people of Fleurance are far from rich and lack many of the luxuries the city dweller takes for granted. In fact, they are by and large indifferent to these luxuries. But they are well aware of their special blessings and want to hold onto them. Hence many of them feel anxious about the insidious changes in the environment that menace the natural order of things. When I spoke to people I noticed that certain problems were mentioned again and again.

People told me: "We are afraid of being poisoned. The water in the canal has turned rank. The same thing is happening to our brooks and ponds."

"We don't know where all the refuse is coming from. The town dump isn't big enough to handle the load. How can we keep down all this rubbish?"

"Our slaughterhouse is antiquated. We're not sure about its sanitary standards. We don't trust the official inspectors. It's important to have good-quality meat."

So it wasn't long before I realized that one of the major tasks of a municipality was to keep down the sources of pollution within its borders. The Society of Environmental Protection had already taken this approach. It had been distributing pamphlets warning the public against certain chemical products that have not yet been officially banned in France but whose harmful effects have been amply demonstrated. More recently the Society had begun to direct its appeals especially to mayors. It was asking them to help educate the public on the environmental question, for this sort of education can best be carried out on the local level. The Society, for instance, had requested mayors to publicize the dangers associated with pesticides and to coordinate efforts within their own communities to keep down the amounts of pesticides used.

Mayors have more power than they imagine. When I was elected mayor of Fleurance in February 1971, the first thing I did was look into the lawbooks. For although I came to the job with great ambitions, I did not want to overstep the boundaries of my office to the slightest degree. It was thus that I discovered that Article 81 of the Administrative Code permitted mayors to make certain rulings by decree. At once it became apparent to me that this authority could be used to excellent effect in the fight against pollution. I would see what I could do with it and how far it would take me.

Unfortunately, most towns lack the funds for any massive antipollution program. Fleurance was no exception. And in a town like ours, where money was hard to come by, it would be doubly difficult to make people give up anything they considered economically beneficial.

As mayor, I had to consider the whole picture seriously. It stood to reason that my town would not be happy if it were not also prosperous. I was duty-bound to look after my people's material well-being as well as after the state of their health. Certainly I couldn't interfere in their economic lives and tell them not to engage in this or that activity because it harmed the environment unless I were ready to offer them a better alternative.

I admit I was baffled for a while.

It is not easy to bring prosperity to a little town with a long past of poverty behind it. Fleurance was almost famous for its poverty. There was a local jingle that went:

> The day when Lectoure's pride will bend,
> And Gimot loses her good wine,
> And Beaumont's bread is not so fine,
> And Fleurance has some sous to spend,
> The world will be close to its end.

Historically, Fleurance has been less fortunate than some of her neighbors, for she was repeatedly struck by famine and pestilence. Yet there was a time in the eighteenth century when her artisans and tradesmen brought considerable wealth into the town. This period lasted into the Napoleonic era, and the town was sufficiently proud of itself to adopt the Latin motto: *Florentia floruit, floret, semperque florabit.* (Fleurance has flowered, is flowering and will forever flower.) But conditions gradually changed and Fleurance once more became a little country town with no outstanding character.

It may seem I am delving far into the past when I should be concentrating on the present-day situation. But I feel that the laws that have presided over the development of a town hold a 'clue to its proper future. In this respect a town is like a human being, whose personality is to a large extent formed in childhood. In order to guide his present, we must understand the individual's past, while remaining faithful to his deeper being.

And so my mind lingered over that old motto—*Florentia floruit, floret, semperque florabit.* Why not take flowers as the starting point of my campaign for the environment? At first my emphasis on flowers made the townspeople smile. "The mayor has a weakness for flowers," they said. My political opponents did not take so forbearing a view. "What about the potholes in the road?" they asked. "And the condition of the town slaughterhouse? And our problems with the water supply? Our tax revenues should go toward sensible things, not foolishness."

But I kept remembering how Fleurance had prided herself on her flowers two centuries ago, and felt she would do well to return to this tradition. Besides, I always urge my patients to have flowers about them. "Keep a flower at your bedside table," I tell them. "It will help you get well." I recommend the same thing to people in good health. "Put flowers on the dinner table," I say. "Whatever you eat, however spare, will taste the better for it." I also think that no one should do without flowers because of lack of money. One may not be able to afford a handsome home, but one can always afford flowers, if only a single bloom at a time. If nothing else, one can always pick a flower from a neighbor's bush, as I myself used to do when I was a penniless boy.

I went on brooding over the town's past. During its most prosperous era it had been something of a commercial center. Well, we might try to stimulate local trade. Most of our shops were located in the arcades that ringed the principal square. Every time I went to my office in the town hall I would pass the merchants' stalls. "How are things going?" I would ask.

"Bah," the shopkeepers would answer. "We just barely make out."

Some would tell me a bit about their problems. "The merchandise isn't what it used to be. Our shop always had a reputation for quality. But nowadays where are you going to get good meat, or fruits and vegetables with any flavor to them? Besides the customers don't know good from bad anymore. All they care about is the appearance of things. They buy with their eyes."

Well, why should the merchants buck the trend? Wasn't it easier to accommodate to the situation? But they would always bridle at this idea. They had their honor as merchants—in the past they had faith in what they sold, and that faith made it easy to open the shop every morning and arrange the wares and exchange a few friendly words with the customers, even though there was not much in the till at the day's end. After all, that wasn't what mattered. In a town like Fleurance, with its five thousand inhabitants, one could not count on getting rich.

"Why not?" I asked.

"Because for a little town to get rich nowadays, it has to have something to offer tourists. Places like Lectoure or Auch are lucky. They have historical features, châteaux, museums, cathedrals. But here there's nothing to attract attention. No one even stops here."

In any case our department of Gers had missed out on the Industrial Revolution, missed out on the canal which was supposed to be dug through the Pyrenées, missed out on railroad connections. So, from one mischance to another, Gers became one of the poorest departments in the country. The proportion of the work force engaged in agriculture—75 percent—is among the highest in the world. And that, any economist will tell you, is no sign of prosperity.

Nevertheless, when I look about the town I am inclined to believe my fellow citizens are wrong to be disheartened about themselves. True, they have been bypassed by progress. But for that very reason they still possess what has become increasingly rare: a sense of happiness. Not far below the surface of their minds is all the robust wisdom of the past, with its appreciation of what it means to be alive. And that, nowadays, is an unusual treasure.

I was discussing the general health of the townspeople with one of my good friends, Dr. Ortholan, who has been practicing medicine at Fleurance for twenty-six years. He confirmed my impression that the people enjoyed unusual longevity and that their constitutions were remarkably strong. "How can you account for this," I asked him, "in view of the effects of modern diet?" For Dr. Ortholan knew and agreed with my theories on the importance of nutrition in keeping people well.

"You must realize," the doctor answered, "that our countryfolk aren't fools. To be sure, they raise their livestock by the usual modern methods, using grain company feeds , with all those chemical additives. But they always raise a few calves for their own use, and these are fed in the good old ways on milk and rich grass, while the hens are allowed to forage in the yard and the family pig receives its bucket of swill morning and night.

"Our country folk work things out pretty well for themselves, I assure you. Part of what they raise is for cash, and there they follow the modern methods that promise them better prices. But another part is for their own table, and there they do things the old way, as their fathers and grandfathers used to. What motivates them is not any concern for nutrition but simply their appreciation of good food."

I began to see that my efforts at environmental reform would be blocked not by any philosophical disagreement, but by the profit motive. That confirmed my earlier feeling that I couldn't ignore people's material interests. But if I could manage to further those interests while also putting across my reforms, all would be well.

So one day shortly after I became mayor I went around to all the butcher shops and *charcuteries* of Fleurance—there are a round dozen of them—and broke my news to the proprietors.

"I'm going to put through new regulations on meat and meat products. From now on no chemical additives and no more doctoring of the meat with preservatives and coloring matter."

My words invariably caused a fluster. "To do that to us, Monsieur Mességué, when we helped elect you! Regulations like that will be our ruin!"

I then explained my program point by point. Above all, I tried to persuade them, they would not lose a *sou*.

"You'll see," I told each of the shopkeepers. "Of course, you'll have to raise prices a bit, but you will be entitled to put a sign in your window: 'Only natural products sold here. Guaranteed pure.' And the customers will come flocking, I promise you. People are ready to pay the difference. I know this for a fact."

"And where are we going to find beef animals that haven't been stuffed with all kinds of artificial rations?" they asked me. "We know of a few farmers who still raise animals by honest methods, but only on a very small scale—not nearly enough to supply the whole town."

"Well, you must pass along word of the new regulations and tell the farmers bluntly that you won't buy their stock unless the animals have been raised naturally. If all twelve of you take that stand, the farmers will have no choice. You'll see, they haven't forgotten how to do it."

"And how will we know they aren't tricking us?"

"You can pay a visit to the farms now and then and see how the animals are being fed. When you've found someone whose methods satisfy you, stick with him and give him preferential prices. And you can also ask him to do what I am going to ask you to do: sign a written agreement that will serve as a warranty."

"You are not going to ask us to do that, Monsieur Mességué?"

"Yes, I am."

On the fifteenth of April, after much grumbling, the twelve shopkeepers of Fleurance delivered their statement to my office in the town hall:

To the Mayor of Fleurance:

In compliance with your appeal, we the undersigned butchers and charcutiers of the town of Fleurance, pledge that we will carry only those meats and meat products which to the best of our knowledge have been raised locally and without the use of artificial rations and chemical substances injurious to the health of the consumer.

Twelve signatures followed in a neat column. Other pledges came in, all obtained by more or less the same approach. There was one from our chief meat dealer, promising to buy only stock raised by wholesome methods. This was the person with whom all our farmers did business and through whom their veal, beef, mutton and pork were distributed to the larger market. His compliance meant my experiment was reaching into a somewhat wider sphere and I was very interested to know what the effect would be. On September 22 the following statement reached my office:

To His Honor the Mayor of Fleurance:

Since we supply the lunchrooms of the Fleurance school system, we guarantee to furnish only milk-fed veal and other meats of certified purity.

This was an important aspect of my program. The new school term was beginning and I did not like to think the children would be exposed to food of doubtful quality. I knew that the meats they were getting at home were wholesome, thanks to the pledges of my butchers. But there is not enough supervision of what goes into school lunches and the newspapers too often carry reports of entire schools being poisoned through the carelessness or dishonesty of the kitchen staff. All in all, it was reassuring to know that in Fleurance, at least, the school lunches would be of a high standard.

By and by interesting notices began appearing in the town's shop windows. The greengrocer advertised: "Organic Fruits and Vegetables," while some of the restaurants added the little slogan: "We Specialize in Natural Products" to their bills of fare. People began to wonder what this was all about. Once they learned the meaning of these new terms, they wondered whether the products were as good as claimed.

I myself could vouch that they were. The vegetables all came from local growers, who upon my urging had begun using barn-yard manures and compost in place of chemical fertilizers. As for the town's best restaurant, as a lover of good food I now and then treated myself to a meal there and knew what went on in its kitchen. The cooking was done by the owner and his wife, who would greet me and recommend some of the Gascon specialties —the rabbit stew or the smoked goose, the pigeon pies or the restaurant's own *pâté*. I would sometimes go down the cellar with the owner and see him draw wine from the cask. I knew that the rabbit had been raised only a few doors away and had been fed on clover and oats, not on commercial rabbit pellets. In fact, I had sometimes seen the restaurant owner's wife carry a basket full of potato peels and bits of bread to the neighbor's and return holding a rabbit by its ears. The line between producer and consumer could hardly be more direct.

I knew that other foods served by the restaurant came from a nearby farm, which also supplied the pork that went into the *pâté*. The poultry there were raised on pure grain, without any additives, while the pigs were fattened on the miscellaneous leftovers of the farming operation—surplus fruit, sour milk, undersized potatoes. The animals did not grow so fast but their meat was lean and tasty.

I knew that at harvest time the restaurant owner went to a certain vintner a few kilometers from Fleurance to stock his cellar for the year. The two men had done business together for a long time and the restaurant owner took as keen an interest as the grower in the summer's weather and the ripening of the grapes. Some years were better than others, but on the whole he could be sure that this country wine had been made of healthy fruit pressed with care, aged with patience and sold without fanfare to local people for a reasonable price. It was not a great wine perhaps, but it captured the mellowness of the sun and the chalkiness of our local soil and could be drunk freely without the slightest regrets. No additives had gone into the cask.

But although small shopkeepers and modest restaurants can keep a sharp eye on the quality of the products they offer, large businesses are too far removed from their source of supply to do so. That is why I am particularly proud of one aspect of our experiment in Fleurance, for we managed to enlist the town su-permarket in our crusade.

Louis Gilles, proprietor of the Alpha supermarket, is a well-in-formed man who is himself a believer in natural foods. I did not have to convince him to join our ranks for he was quite eager to do so, although he imagined that the wholesalers would give him endless trouble. My only role was to encourage him and join him in rejoicing over the victories, which proved to be more nu-merous than he had expected. Each time I dropped in at the supermarket, Louis Gilles had some new letters to show me.

"Have a look at this one," he would say. And I would read:

> We the packagers of Chicory X guarantee that our product contains nothing but pure ground chicory root, roasted for optimum flavor. No chemical substance of any sort has gone into its preparation.

Another letter from a local preserves firm certified:

> We hereby declare that all the jams and jellies shipped to the Alpha supermarket in Fleurance are made of nothing but pure fruit and sugar, and are free of coloring matter or chemical preservatives.

Even more significant was a letter from Louis Gilles' chief sup-plier of milk products:

> We of the Cooperative Dairy take pride in the fact that all our yogurts, custards, soft cheeses and creams are made of pure whole milk without the addition of any chemical preserva-tives.

Another firm boasted of its continuous concern with sanitary standards:

> We maintain our own laboratory which makes a daily check of the freshness and cleanliness of our products. All the stan-dards set by the Board of Health are rigorously observed.

All in all, the picture seemed better than we had counted on. "Have all the answers been so encouraging?" I asked Gilles.

"Not at all," he said. "Some of the suppliers simply refuse to answer my inquiry, or to give me any kind of gurantee."

"What can you do about them?" I asked.

"I can simply send my orders elsewhere."

"How can you know that the firms that give you written guarantees aren't faking?"

"They would hardly do that," he answered. "These matters can easily be checked and I could make trouble for them later. Some of the suppliers simply decide to let me have their pure products and channel the rest elsewhere. For instance, they send me their unflavored and fruit yogurt, while the kind with artificial coloring, which always has plenty of takers, goes to all the other retailers. So they are not really inconvenienced by our desire to observe these standards."

The various certifications were posted on a bulletin board at the supermarket and the customers would cluster around and consult the list before setting off to fill their baskets. Some of the statements came from makers of well-known brands who were secure in their position, while others were handwritten letters from small local producers who took personal pride in declaring the purity of their honey, their eggs and their chicken.

At the meat department of the supermarket the Soubirous, father and son, kept a sharp eye on the quality of the meat they offered—a rare situation in supermarkets. They had put up a little notice: "Our veal is all milk-fed."

I always stopped to have a word with them, for I had gone to school with the older Soubirous. This time I asked about the notice: "How can you be sure that your veal was milk-fed?"

"That's easy. When I go to the farms to do my buying, I always look to see how many calves they have around. If there are just two or three gamboling in the nearest field, then I know that the animals are being raised on milk. But if it's a large-scale operation, I know it's just the opposite."

I kept a daily watch over the progress of the campaign in Fleurance. I had promised everybody higher profits if they kept faith with me. Since everyone had had to raise prices a little, this was a tricky matter.

"How is business going?" I asked as I strolled about town.

The supermarket was in the midst of a boom. "My volume has about doubled," Louis Gilles told me. "People are coming from some distance, from Rabastens, from Agen and even from Toulouse to do their grocery shopping in Fleurance."

The butcher shops and *charcuteries* were also doing well.

"Well, Maurice, I'm making you a present of a ham," one of my most reluctant signers told me.

"A present from you, the stingiest man in Fleurance!" I exclaimed.

"You will remember, I didn't think much of your campaign at the beginning," he said. "But nowadays business is so good I can't keep up with the demand."

One day toward the end of the summer I dropped in at the *charcuterie* located on the other side of the market square opposite the town hall. I was surprised at how bare it looked.

"Have you been burgled?" I asked.

"No, I've been sold out," the owner answered. "We're had so many tourists that I'm all out of hams and sausages. I'm closing up for a few weeks and going on vacation with my wife. We haven't had a holiday in years and years."

This news pleased me all the more because the owner had been one of the leaders of the anti-Messegué faction and a vociferous member of the town government.

Everywhere I went I heard the same thing. "Your Honor, the tourists were a real plague this summer, worse than grasshoppers. They bought up everything. We can't find a ham anywhere in town. The tobacco shop is clean out of postcards of Fleurance."

Once the Fleurantins realized they were on to a good thing, they went to work with a will. A group of the more dynamic citizens came to me to discuss a new venture. "We want to start a line of natural products," they said, "under the brand name of *Fleurance*. We'll test and recommend products and distribute them with our label. Of course, we'll specialize in local products but we'll also include things from elsewhere if they conform to our standards."

In the autumn of 1971 the "Fleurance" brand was launched. It offered a wide range of foodstuffs, from Norwegian charcoal-smoked salmon to an assortment of mountain honeys from all over Europe, from country wines of guaranteed purity to hams cured by old-fashioned methods that brought out all their flavor.

Often the director of the new company, Jean-Jacques Castel, would invite me to a sampling, though I had had no actual part in the enterprise. "We want your opinion on a couple of items," he would say. "Do they deserve to have our label?" For it was not enough for a product to conform to standards of purity. It had also to meet the highest standards of gastronomy. Gascony, after all, has a certain tradition to maintain.

I was very pleased at how well the venture was going for it seemed heartening evidence that my theories were practical. Castel kept me informed of the latest developments.

"The orders come pouring in," he told me. "We have contracts with hundreds of health food stores in France and abroad. But we are running into a serious problem."

"What is that?"

"A matter of supply. We are scouring the countryside for good wholesome products but there are simply not enough being grown. You will have to help us, Maurice."

"In what way?"

"Try to convince the farmers that it would be worth their while to aim for quality. They seem to have a lot of reservations about it."

So I offered to accompany my friend Castel on one of his scouting trips. He was going to see a farmer that very day and we drove out to what was obviously a thriving place run on efficient lines. Castel and the farmer began their discussion while I stood by with paper and pencil. Soon we were deep in figures, computing bushels and labor costs very much as in those arithmetic problems children are set at school.

"How much do you generally clear on an acre of wheat?" Castel asked.

The farmer named a sum.

"You have that down, Maurice? All right. Now suppose you converted that acre into tomatoes for us. Since you'll be growing them the organic way, you can leave out the expense of chemical fertilizer and sprays . . ."

We did some more figuring, considering average yields and harvesting costs.

"Suppose I guaranteed to buy those tomatoes at so much a bushel—how much would you clear?"

Again we plunged into involved computations. The final figure was considerably higher than the one for wheat and the farmer's attitude was far less suspicious than it had been at the beginning.

"What I'd like to do is draw up a written agreement," Castel said, "and if you're satisfied with the way it goes, we can make it two acres next year."

The experiment had a happy outcome, with the farmer realizing even larger returns than he had anticipated. We weren't asking him to revolutionize his habits from one day to the next. Just one acre of tomatoes. Or just one litter of piglets. Just one brood of ducklings. Just a few crates of berries. On this basis we had no trouble signing contracts.

In our search for organically-grown products we were fortunate to receive the wholehearted backing of our regional agricultural bureau. The new firm could not as yet send out its own team of inspectors but the agricultural bureau offered to check on the methods used and to give the farmers enrolled in our program whatever technical guidance they required—for the farmers had become so dependent on chemical products of one kind or another that they no longer knew how to operate without them. But with good advice from the bureau they were evidently so successful that by the end of 1971 a group of Fleurance farmers had formed a cooperative to sell their organically-grown products directly to the retailer. My town was becoming national headquarters for the movement for wholesome food.

The movement, however, could not long be confined. Soon the town of Valence d'Agen, in the department of Tarn-et-Garonne, was instituting an interesting practice. Under the leadership of its mayor, Mme. Baylet, who is also the owner of the newspaper *Dépêche du Midi*, the town had divided its poultry market into two sections: one side devoted to chickens, ducks, turkeys and geese raised on a large scale with modern feeds, and the other side selling fowl raised on a diet of basic grains. I was so struck by this idea that I introduced it to Fleurance. Now our poultry market is similarly divided, with the two sides clearly marked. Only when the consumer knows what he is being offered is he in a position to make his choice. I was not surprised that the demand for the fowls raised on simple grain free of any additives was considerably larger than for the others.

When I was elected vice president of the National Association of Mayors, I felt I ought to tell my colleagues about these experiments in the hope that other regions might want to introduce similar measures adapted to local conditions. Soon I was being invited to speak at towns all over France to describe what we had been doing at Fleurance. Meanwhile, the same call was being issued elsewhere, for the urgency of our situation was widely felt, though people did not yet know what methods could be devised to make the necessary transformation a reality. Yet certain ideas were already in the air. Thus one speaker before the Rouen branch of the Society of Environmental Protection made the prediction: "The smaller French towns will lead the way in offering people a better mode of life." That was very much the line I was following and I was increasingly convinced that it was a fruitful one.

My hope has been that our activities in Fleurance will serve as a sort of pilot project to demonstrate that towns can take the initiative in reversing the dangerous trends toward pollution. They can do this, moreover, without depending on government funds, while at the same time revitalizing their economies. This lesson has special meaning for the so-called poor regions of France. The traditionally rich regions such as Brie and Beauce are admirably suited for large-scale agriculture and will continue to produce in quantity. But we in other regions can develop a different sort of agriculture, where personal responsibility and concern for quality are the primary factors.

Our aim is to make conversions, among both consumers and producers, and restore values that were normal not too long ago but were lost in the race for maximum yields and quick profits. For we have become disillusioned with these short-term goals. The contemporary world is looking for something quite different. In terms of food, we are looking for savor and soundness. In terms of existence, are we not looking for much the same?

Our department of Gers is a good example of what I mean. Its forested hills produce vast quantities of refreshing ozone. As the air of the cities and the industrialized areas grows increasingly polluted, we begin to appreciate what clean air means. We begin to see that it is not something to be taken for granted but represents a vital resource. Gers and places like it must be considered a reservoir for the rest of the country. And not for air only. The countryside, unmarred by industry and blatant commerce, is lovely to the eye and soothing to the heart. Here people still have time to tend their flowers, their home vegetable gardens and their fruit trees. Here planting and harvesting retain their old meaning —for what we sow, whether good or bad, we shall surely reap.

I believe it is urgent to find and preserve such islands of tranquility throughout the world where people can catch their breath from the dizzy race of progress. Just as any city, to be livable, has to preserve its surrounding green belts, its parks and its little squares, so every country must jealously guard its wilderness areas, its mountains, forests and heaths, and its farming regions as well, particularly those where time-honored methods are still followed.

Economists may label such districts as poor. To me, they are far richer than industrialized areas, for they supply something that cannot be measured in tonnage or annual sales figures: happiness.

I am not advocating that we turn back the clock and abandon all twentieth-century contributions to agriculture. Our Fleurance products are scarcely going to feed the whole nation, especially with the increasing demand for more meat, more dairy products. Our organically-raised foods represent only one choice among many others. But just as the salons of *haute couture* exist alongside ordinary garment manufacturing and offer a degree of leadership in the creation of fashion, so organically-raised food has its place and its mission within the framework of our national agriculture. By setting standards of taste and nutrition it can raise the entire level of agricultural production.

Statistics tell us that from year to year the average family spends proportionately less of its income on food. The percentage devoted to housing, clothing and leisure time activities has increased. We have better homes, we dress better, we seek out more amusements. Some of us might choose to allocate a bit more of our budget to purer food, especially when we know that our health and that of our family will benefit thereby.

Speaking of the uses of the family budget, I would like to make another suggestion. I firmly believe that everyone needs an emotional attachment to some bit of the country, that in the absence of such a link he is not really complete. Many city dwellers are fortunate enough to have a grandmother, an old aunt or some good friends who live in country districts and in whose homes they are welcome guests. Others may have a vacation place or country cottage where they mean to spend their retirement years.

But I would urge families that lack such retreats to search out some part of the country that appeals to them and make it the place where they customarily go. A vacation spent in a single spot is always more restorative than the same amount of time spent in restless touring. Small villages are attractive places to stay. They cost less than the crowded seaside or mountain resorts and offer rich terrain for private discoveries. The children of the family will look forward to returning to a familiar landscape filled with rich association, for them. For nature reveals secrets to a child that remain unforgotten in later years. Children, even more than adults, quickly form those thousand tiny bonds with trees and flowers and sky and farm animals by which human beings achieve a relationship to the earth. Adults also benefit by the natural pulse of country life. The quiet days bring an inner renewal to our bodies and spirits, otherwise battered by the artificial excitements of our times.

The tourist bureaus are always helpful in finding accommodations. In many parts of the country, camping facilities on private farms are available.

Through such vacations a new sort of friendship will grow up between city people and country people. I would dearly wish for a reconciliation between these two groups. They have been long estranged and at the moment seem hardly to be speaking the same language. Each regards the other as something of an enemy, whereas in fact they should recognize their mutual dependence. The city man should know that there would be no food on his table without the labors of the country man, while the farmer should understand that the city people of whom he speaks with scorn represent his major market. Acquaintanceship would break down these barriers. The city man is by no means as stuck-up as the farmer thinks him. To be sure, he always wears a necktie, but behind that facade of dignity he has far more uncertainties about himself than the country man can even imagine. He suffers in ways the country man is spared. I can see some of this when he comes to me as a patient. Sunlight makes him squint and the slightest breeze makes him shiver. When I tell him to go out in the fields and gather flowers, he blushes like a schoolboy, so shy is he in the presence of nature.

As for the country dweller, he has his complexes, too. He has kept contact with things of the earth, but he feels awkward when he has to step outside his village. When country-born young people leave the land, the rupture causes more psychic damage than is generally recognized. They break not only with their families but also with ways of feeling for which they do not easily find a substitute. There is a hollowness in them and they do not know how to fill it. When they revisit their native villages it is in most cases to show off their success.

Thus bit by bit the gulf between country dweller and city dweller has widened. I would like to bridge this gulf and bring each group to a better understanding of the other. This book is an attempt to do so. The time for rediscovery has come, and both sides will gain immeasurably from it. The city dweller will recover health and happiness, the country dweller will find regeneration and dignity.

3. Cultivate Your Garden

*May death find me planting my
cabbages, indifferent to his threat
and even more so to my garden's
imperfections.*

I borrow a maxim from Montaigne. The same image occurs in a centuries-old game of French children, where they mimic the actions of planting cabbages, walking an imaginary path and stooping to drop seeds into an imaginary furrow *à la mode de chez nous.*

Montaigne would sometimes desert his study for the kitchen garden where he would look after his cabbages and presumably the other vegetables he had planted there. The essayist had great respect for the humble tasks of life. Voltaire's hero Candide also took refuge from unanswerable questions in tending his garden. Unfortunately, twentieth-century man seldom has a garden he can step into. He is surrounded by sidewalks and these do not promote the cultivation of a personal philosophy.

I would like to see kitchen gardens revived on a large scale. I would urge everyone who lives in the country or has a second home there to devote a small plot to some vegetables and health-giving herbs. A flower garden lends great charm to a house, delighting the eye and the sense of smell. But behind the house there is always room for at least a few rows of salad material. If you live in an apartment, of course, acquiring a patch of soil is harder. But it is worth giving up a month's vacation at the seashore and devoting the money to buying an allotment strip on the outskirts of town. The pleasure of working there on weekends will more than make up for the sacrifice. Moreover, the yield of even the smallest plot of ground, if well managed, is surprising. In a few seasons your harvests will make up for the initial cost.

Commercial agriculture is dependent on chemical fertilizers and insecticides. But the small garden can do without these. If you raise vegetables for your family the organic way, you can be confident that your produce will be of higher nutritional value than anything you can buy. Make use of manures and mulches. You can also apply potash, lime and sulphur in small quantities, but beware of any of the synthetic mixtures. You are not aiming for maximum quantity, after all, but for superior flavor.

Read a few good gardening books, preferably older ones, which explain the secrets of the soil, the propitious times for sowing and the influence of the phases of the moon. If you have already tried growing flowers or indoor plants and have proved to have something of a green thumb, your vegetable seeds will not fail you either. Your cabbages will be as plump as your roses are beautiful.

Decide how much area you want to allow for the basic vegetables: carrots, cabbage, tomatoes, lettuce, garlic, onion, celery, leeks. If your space is limited, you had better rule out potatoes. Perhaps you will have room for some dwarf fruit trees, strawberries, current bushes, a selection of herbs, and in a quiet corner why not install a beehive?

A well cared for vegetable plot with its neat beds and straight rows is as pleasant to behold as a formal garden. But nature has her rules—which are not entirely the same as those of landscape architects. When nettles spring up at the foot of your hedge, they give the garden a somewhat rough look. But you would be wrong to weed them out, for somehow their presence makes any fragrant herbs growing nearby more pungent.

There are many such mysterious relationships among plants which should be respected. Certain vegetables have clear affinities for each other and thrive when planted side by side. Examples of such natural partnerships are onions and beets, leeks and celery, carrots and peas, tomatoes and parsley. Others, however, are antagonistic: tomatoes and fennel, tomatoes and kohlrabi. A number of vegetables are highly impressionable and take on the taste of their neighbors. This is especially true of radishes. A bed of radishes bordered by four different vegetables will give you radishes of four distinct flavors. The proximity of garden cress seems to bring out the best in radishes. Chervil makes them overly sharp, while if the radishes are planted quite by themselves, they will be too bland.

Be careful not to plant your fruit trees and berry bushes too close to your vegetable plot or else the vegetables will be shaded out. Vegetables require full sun. Here and there about the edges you will want to include a patch of mint, a few geraniums, a border of nasturtiums, a row of onions and a dozen tomato plants. Since you prefer to have nothing to do with chemical sprays and dusts, you must protect your fruits and vegetables with these staunch guardian plants. They all have the power of repelling insects, yet are agreeable and useful in their own right.

Once you have planted your seeds, watch over them with loving care. As soon as they have germinated, study the form of the tiny plants so that you will never mistake them for the weeds that spring up in abundance and have to be plucked out. Water and hoe, thin and transplant, stake and tie. These tasks are all enjoyable in themselves and will assure you a bountiful harvest.

Some years your harvest may seem even too bountiful and you may groan at the prodigality of nature. But remember that summers are short. Make provision for the future, like the proverbial ant. Prepare jams and pickles, learn the techniques of home canning—they are not difficult and your jars of homegrown tomatoes will taste far better than the commercial sort. If, on the other hand, the weather is bad and your garden has been disappointing, learn to make use of the wild plants growing nearby. Young nettles, boiled, make delicious greens. Purslane, which crops up uninvited in cultivated soil and is generally weeded out, is good as a salad or a boiled green. The same is true of dandelion. Nasturtium leaves make spicy salads and garnishes.

Portions of vegetables generally thrown away can be turned to good use. Examples are carrot and radish tops, both of which contribute a distinctive flavor to soups. And remember that a handful of tops from home-grown radishes thrown into the soup kettle is richer in nutriments than the finest of vegetables raised on commercial fertilizer.

Once you have come to appreciate the qualities of plants, you will think up hundreds of ways to prepare them for your family's pleasure. This book offers a group of recipes, some traditional, some new, which indicate how the most modest plants can be turned into delicacies. But before we go into the specifics of cooking, let me emphasize that the good old family soup tureen is worth more than all the medicines in the world. It is truly a fount of health. Alexandre Dumas once described the French as "a soup-eating people." This definition no longer holds. It is a great pity but we French do not depend upon soups as we used to, partly because the housewife no longer can spare the time to prepare her own, partly because other foods have come to take their place.

I would not deny the value of the protein foods (meats, eggs, milk, cheese) but our forbears always set great store by vegetables, and with good reason. Many vegetables, while low in calories (a virtue, from the contemporary point of view), are very high in vitamins of all sorts. And vitamins, although a modern discovery, have always been indispensable to life. Vegetables, in fact, have actual medicinal properties of which we ought to be aware.

Unfortunately modern medicine, in its pride over its remarkable advances, tends to disparage the "old wives'" recipes that once enjoyed high favor. The pharmocopeia of the twentieth century has indeed wonderful resources at its command, but all these new drugs are expensive and often produce dangerous side effects. Yet nature has furnished us with a host of harmless and efficacious remedies that cost almost nothing. A licensed pharmacist who stands behind his counter in a white jacket would feel it far beneath his dignity to give his customer carrots, cabbage and parsley. "You have come to the wrong shop," he would say. "The greengrocer is down the street." Nevertheless, the great pharmaceutical houses will occasionally market an extract of garlic, or a syrup of ivy or myrtle. One celebrated Dutch drug company has put out capsules whose chief ingredient is cabbage juice. In fact, more of the products at the druggist's are based on vegetable extracts than the public realizes.

Human vanity plays a part in this. To be sure, Hippocrates, the father of medicine, maintained that there were certain sicknesses that could be treated only by diet. But what self-respecting doctor, even if he were convinced of the virtues of certain vegetables, would dare to prescribe such homely measures to his patients? He has to use terms that look impressive on a prescription slip. The patient, too, might feel insulted at being told by his doctor to eat a dish of carrots every evening, or a good bowl of cabbage soup at noon.

The patient wants above all to have his ailments taken seriously. He has come to think that the efficacy of a medicine must be proportional to its price. This is a misconception fostered by the publicity given to modern wonder drugs. There are, of course, new drugs that are prodigiously expensive and can work miracles. But there are also remedies that cost almost nothing and are nevertheless highly efficacious.

In Russia, where folk medicine has retained a place alongside conventional medicine, the picture is totally different. There medicine is unaffected by the profit motive and the pharmaceutical laboratories are owned and supported by the state. Under such conditions old-style healers do not represent dangerous competition to the medical profession. On the contrary, their lore is valued and often used as a base for present-day research.

Soviet pharmacies are run along austere lines. There is no advertising or fancy packaging. No effort is made to increase consumption of any item. The objective is to offer simple but sound drugs that can be dispensed on a nationwide scale. No glamor attaches to the latest discovery. Only the results count. The level of health in the Soviet Union has risen dramatically in the past half-century and life expectancy has greatly increased. Throughout the country medical research is held in high esteem.

Nevertheless, the Soviet people have retained their faith in simple remedies. According to an old Russian saying: "Anyone who understands nature never need be sick." I myself share this view. If people knew the blessings contained in each round cabbage growing in their gardens, they could watch over it as over a treasure and eat of it with deep respect. For vegetables can keep us well all our lives, and if by some mischance some minor troubles should interfere with our organic functioning, the proper use of vegetables can right the matter and restore the body's equilibrium in short order.

Vegetables are looked upon as common and hence somewhat crude. This is hardly so. As plants, they are shortlived but nonetheless highly developed organisms. Their past stretches back to the earliest cultures of mankind. How carefully their seeds must have been gathered and preserved from harvest to harvest! With what piety must they have been carried from the mother country to the new colonies, or collected by travelers and soldiers and brought back from foreign parts as valuable curiosities. How much attention must have been paid to their requirements, long before the age of scientific selection and experimental stations. Their history is not the less illustrious for having gone unrecorded.

Like human beings, vegetables should not be judged solely by their appearance. Some of the most delicious kinds are drab-looking. The smaller variety may be far superior in quality to the heavy-bearer developed for commercial use. The fanciest specimen may be deficient in flavor. Your home-grown tomato may not be a perfect globe, your lettuce may be darker green and more wrinkled than the hothouse product, but your salad will taste the better for these idiosyncrasies.

Apples from your own trees may be scabby, but do not think less of them for that. Their rough skin is frequently the promise of a more·fragrant fruit than any you can buy. Their color is indubitably finer. Certainly they are far better for you than fruits that have been saturated with insecticides, hormone sprays and ripening agents. Since you cannot sell them, keep them for your family's own use. There are so many ways to treat apples that not a single one should go to waste. Bottle the surplus as apple sauce and apple butter and you will have their goodness all year round. Of all fruits, apples are particularly healthful.

It would not be too difficult, I think, to bring unsprayed fruit back into favor. Their minor blemishes could be accepted as part of their charm. After all, our current crop of starlets have made a selling point of the freckles that were the despair of their grandmothers. As a result, many girls will use an eyebrow pencil to dot some freckles on their noses—which marks a strange reversal from the former demand for porcelain-clear complexions. On the other hand, we may recall that there were periods when women adorned their faces with so-called patches and painted beauty marks.

So does the wheel of fashion turn and it is human nature to try to conform to each of its revolutions. The day may come when we will see apples and pears displayed for sale with the odd-shaped and speckled ones on top. I would not mind inspiring such a movement. Fashions, however capricious they may seem at first glance, are motivated by a need to right the balance. The day when the housewife looks tenderly upon a knobby apple or a rough-skinned pear will mark the end of the false ideal of the perfect fruit, which in most cases has neither taste nor texture to commend it. Then people will choose their fruit for its real character and not for its outward appearance. They will remember how good the old varieties tasted, and just as battered trunks are the ones which contain treasures and dented kettles make the most savory stews, so the gnarled fruit trees in grandmother's garden will be rediscovered. Horticulturists will turn to these old trees, just when they are in danger of dying out, and propagate a host of saplings from them. And we will once more bite into apples with true enjoyment.

Let us take a stroll through one of those kitchen gardens of yesteryear and go from bed to bed, communing with the various vegetables. For there is wisdom in them, along with nourishment.

Garlic

Let us begin with garlic, which I as a Gascon hold very dear and which occupies an important place in my system of therapy. In fact, I can hardly say whether I value it more for its contribution to good eating or for its medicinal qualities.

For me, garlic is synonymous with vitality. In Gascony we say that we baptize our children by rubbing a clove of garlic on their tongues and following that up with a swallow of armagnac. Then they are ready to meet whatever challenges life brings.

It is well known that Henri IV was baptized in this manner, and mindful of tradition he would meet any challenging moment by chewing a clove of garlic and washing it down with armagnac. These challenging moments for our good King Henri tended to be connected with ladies, and since there were many ladies in his life, he must have chewed many a clove of garlic in his day.

Certain inveterate skirt-chasers in my part of the country,

taking good King Henri as their model, have been known to chew garlic from morning to night to keep themselves in form for their exploits. I remember a certain cavalry officer who used to strut about our town wafting the smell of garlic a hundred feet in all directions. Yet what a reputation he had among the women! His rivals were all furious with envy. He lived, moreover, to a ripe old age.

Often, when I have sought the secret of certain men's vitality, I find the answer lies in garlic. The same is true for animals. Once, when I was on a trip to the West Indies, I was told about a local miracle man who was even more famous for his fighting cocks than for his magical cures. I went to see him out of curiosity. He was very cordial and invited me to spend Christmas Day with him. I could not approve of some of his barbarous practices. "I have killed many men," he freely admitted to me, "but it is only the bad ones who die."

Moreover, I do not care for cockfighting. I have too much respect for animals to enjoy seeing them exploited to minister to the human instinct for cruelty. Nevertheless, I have always been impressed by the astonishing pugnacity of fighting cocks. The miracle man performed some sort of ritual for me, accompanied by the weirdest sounds, which was supposed to make his team of cocks invulnerable. I watched with the greatest interest, wondering what else this miracle man had in his repertory.

"Bah," he said suddenly, "you're not a competitor. You know nothing about cockfighting, and besides, you live too far away. I'm going to show you how I raise my champions."

He led me into a small shed close to his house. It contained several baskets of garlic.

"I put this into their feed," he told me. "About half and half. But you must not tell anyone."

I wanted to laugh. So this was the miracle-man's great secret! The West Indian cocks owed their famous fighting spirit (as did our Gascon cock Henri IV) to garlic! I hope the miracle man will forgive me for revealing his method and not put an evil spell on me. After all, a long time has gone by since he took me into his confidence. Moreover, I have learned through later reading that the Romans used to give their fighting cocks garlic and that the work forces that built the pyramids in ancient Egypt were issued garlic as an important part of their diet. I have invented nothing new in prescribing garlic for my athlete patients—runners, bicyclists and others.

Garlic, then, has its place in history as well as in geography. Significantly, wherever garlic grows (and it is found in most parts of the globe), it is credited with miraculous virtues. In certain regions of the Soviet Union famous for the longevity of their inhabitants, people drink a potion made of garlic juice. The folk doctors recommend a special cure with this product. The garlic is chopped fine and set to steep in alcohol, in proportions of one part garlic to two parts alcohol, The bottle is kept in full sunlight for fifteen days. The liquor is strained and the cure begins with two or three drops taken in a glass of warm water before dinner. Each day the dose is increased until one is taking twenty-five drops, then it is reduced day by day until one is down to a single drop. This cure can be repeated several times in the course of a year, allowing intervals of some weeks between each bout.

Another prescription is to mince two or three cloves of garlic in a glass of white wine, let it steep for a few days and take a teaspoonful of this mixture every morning before breakfast.

But the most pleasant way to take garlic is in food—provided you like the taste. We in the Midi use it liberally and have many recipes in which garlic figures prominently. We even make a soup for babies based on stewed garlic, which acts as an antiworm measure. In the old days a few garlic cloves would be hung around children's necks to ward off intestinal worms. I have heard that it was most effective.

I would advise giving children their garlic by rubbing some energetically over a good crusty piece of country bread, then dripping a bit of olive oil over the slice. This makes an excellent snack for youngsters. I feasted on this all through my childhood. With a bit of salt and a cluster of golden-skinned, sun-warmed grapes, it makes a wonderful lunch.

Garlic is good for you any way you eat it. Those who find it too strong might try the pink variety, or Spanish garlic, whose flavor is more delicate. They can also cut away the germ section, which is especially rich in alliatic acid, the element responsible for "garlic breath."

Perhaps you like garlic but think it interferes with your romantic and social life. In that case it is good to know that a pinch of parsley or a few coffee beans, chewed after eating, will absorb the garlic smell. You might also restrict yourself to eating it only at your evening meal, before going to bed—provided your spouse does not object.

Nowadays an extract of garlic is available at the pharmacy. For a vegetable to be made into a medicament is equivalent to its receiving the Legion of Honor, the culmination of a career of good and loyal service. My friend Garlic has been elevated to the highest rank. I am glad for him, for he deserves the distinction on many counts.

Besides garlic's properties as a vermifuge and tonic, it is also a laxative, diuretic, antiseptic, antibacterial agent, a good resolvent and febrifuge. It contains powerful antibiotic elements. Its sulphur content makes it an excellent pulmonary antiseptic. In bygone times, during epidemics of the plague, doctors would wear masks saturated with garlic juice when visiting the sick. Nowadays statistics indicate that those parts of the world where garlic is eaten in quantity have a low incidence of cancer. Of course, one might point out that these regions are also poor and agricultural, hence less troubled by industrial pollution and chemically treated food.

My own statistics are perhaps too scanty to be adduced as proof. But I have made an observation which I hereby offer in good faith:

Wherever I found garlic in use, I found health.

Conversely, wherever I found healthy people, I found that they were garlic eaters.

Therefore, I coaxed my cousin Michel Descamps into planting an acre of top-quality garlic on his Gavarret farm. I always enlist Michel in my agricultural experiments. Like any canny farmer, he made some calculations before giving me his answer.

"You know, Maurice, if I grow this garlic without chemical fertilizer and herbicides, I'll have to ask about twenty or thirty percent more for it. The yield will be lower and I'll have to put in a lot more weeding and hoeing time."

"Well, that's how it'll have to be, Michel. I think we ought to have some organic garlic to sell, at least in Fleurance. You can also count on orders from Castel. Altogether, we'll take all you can grow and I bet next year you'll be putting in not one acre but two."

I was already imagining the crates of good garlic we would be shipping off in all directions, even to foreign countries, along with recipes for those poor benighted people who wouldn't know what to do with it. Why not pack the pretty garlic bulbs in little boxes, like chocolate bonbons? A box of these would make a charming Christmas present, much better than the usual indigestible and fattening confections. For the moment, of course, this is only a dream. But I mean to go to work on the idea. So do not be surprised if one of these years you find a beribboned box of garlic under the Christmas tree. Don't think it is a practical joke. Rather say: "Here is a friend who cares about me."

Onion

The onion is first cousin to garlic. The two have many qualities in common, so they may be used in place of each other in cooking.

Onion is milder than garlic and the red onion milder still. Unlike many vegetables which lose some of their virtues in cooking, cooked onions are rich in vitamins. But they should not be fried. Add them to stews or bake them. If you like them raw, you may eat them freely that way. I knew one Tour de France champion who would eat a raw onion at each of his stops in the course of the race. He was in his fifties when he consulted me on some of his problems. He would recount his athletic triumphs of the past and would always add: "For me, onion is like dynamite. All I have to do is eat an onion and I'm off like a bombshell."

A boxer has also told me that he "fueled up" with onion.

My farmer neighbors always take a large onion out to the fields with them during the periods of heavy work: planting, haying, harvesting. They eat the onion with a heel of bread during their rest periods and claim it gives them extra energy.

The onion is also credited with aphrodisiac qualities. Onion soup is a favorite dish with night owls and is supposed to prime them for all sorts of adventures. I cannot vouch for this. I do know that onions are conducive to love insofar as they do wonders for women's complexions. And here the ladies are in a quandary. Of course, they want to have lovely skin but how awful to smell of onions! But let them take comfort. Today there are many lozenges based on mint for sweetening the breath. Or, as with garlic, they can nibble some parsley or coffee beans. Meanwhile, there is great satisfaction in watching one's skin improve, eruptions disappear, and in knowing that the intestinal lining is undergoing a similar process. In addition, onion destroys intestinal parasites and can correct various forms of constipation.

Onion is also a good diuretic which acts against retention of fluids and cleanses the system of urea and sodium. Even used externally, onion promotes elimination. Thus one has only to rub the loins with half an onion to increase urination by 25 percent. Such onion massage is also helpful in cases of sciatica.

Eaten raw, onion promotes transpiration and cleanses the pores as effectively as a good sauna bath. Raw onion is especially recommended for rheumatic patients.

Onion extracts are useful against both colds and tonsilitis. Here is an old recipe for concocting one's own "onion wine":

Mix 100 to 150 grams of grated onion with 100 grams of honey. Place in a quart jar and cover with a good white wine. Let the mixture steep for two weeks, then strain. Take three or four spoonfuls of this compound every day. Its taste is somewhat unusual but its effect is highly diuretic and strengthening.

To sum up its powers, onion is a stimulant, a disinfectant and a diuretic. It is effective against intestinal worms, scurvy and rheumatism. Like garlic, it is an excellent antibiotic. Recently it has been found to have antidiabetic properties, inasmuch as it lowers the sugar content in the blood. English scientists have discovered that onion is an effective anticoagulant. Onion may thus turn out to be a powerful weapon in the battle against cardiovascular diseases. In fact, French horse-breeders would seem to have had an instinctive knowledge of this property of the onion, for they have always fed onions to stallions with a tendency toward thrombosis.

All in all, the onion's list of honors is so long that, like garlic, it may be considered among the foremost of the health-giving vegetables.

The other plants of the allium family—leeks, shallots, scallions, chives—have much the same properties but to a lesser degree. Use them liberally, either cooked, as in leek soup, or minced raw in salads. They are milder in taste than the onion and less apt to make you cry. But consider whether you would not gladly weep for a minute or two while peeling your onions if that enables you to laugh heartily your whole life long, in full possession of your health.

Now and then patients and readers write to tell me about an experience of theirs that confirms and supplements my own discoveries. Recently I received a letter from Mme. E.G. of Lavrester, Morbihan, describing still another use of onions. I quote the significant passages:

> In your book *Of Men and Plants* I found no mention of a treatment with which perhaps you are well acquainted. We have relied on it for many years, my father having learned it from an Angevin "sawbones." It involves using onions as a poultice against typhoid.
>
> In previous times, seventy years ago, when my native city of Lorient was surrounded by marshes, typhoid used to be endemic there. Most natives were fairly resistant to it but the fever could be fatal to newcomers. However, we used to treat it with a poultice made of onions. More people were saved by this treatment than I can tell.
>
> This was the procedure. We would take about two kilograms of large onions and chop them fine. These would be spread on a thin linen cloth which we would then wrap around the feet of the patient. The wrapping would remain on overnight, or for a period of eight hours. It was important to protect the bed with a rubber sheet, first because the poultice itself would produce a good deal of moisture and secondly because its diuretic effects could be beyond the patient's control. Within three days the sickness would be past. There were only two cases where the treatment failed—my sister and one of her sons, and it is likely that what they had was not typhoid, though the doctor diagnosed it as such at the time. This was thirty-five years ago. We were acquainted with Dr. D., then director of the Naval Hospital. I told him about our onion poultice. Far from laughing at it, he tried it out at the hospital and as long as he remained director, cases of typhoid fever were given the "onion treatment." I also remember an incident of fifty years ago, when the little daughter of the stationmaster at Lorient

was stricken with scarlet fever and her life was despaired of. My father had the idea of trying the onion poultice and it was marvelously effective.

No doubt I am telling you nothing new. These are only some examples in which you might be interested.

Cabbage

One of the oldest of cultivated vegetables (it was grown as far back as 2000 B.C.), cabbage dominates the kitchen garden by its size, and like every good king, it is also generous. A steaming hot cabbage soup is a great comfort in bitter weather. Such a soup has been known to resuscitate the dying. Country folk like a plate of cabbage soup before leaving for their day's work in the fields.

In Gascony the morning greeting is: "*Adichats, as dejunat?*" or: "Hi! Have you eaten?" Which means: "Have you a good soup in your innards?" The better to fortify ourselves for the hours that lie ahead, we add a dollop of red wine to the last bit of soup in our bowl. There is even a Gascon expression for this: *faire chabrot*.

For some delicate stomachs cooked cabbage is hard to digest. But it is only when boiled that cabbage presents a problem. It is harmless when steamed, or better still, eaten raw in salads. Of course, raw cabbage calls for energetic chewing but it is well worth the trouble. You can also avail yourself of modern technology and put your cabbage through an electric juicer. With a few drops of lemon juice, this makes a delicious drink with the same health-giving properties as the cabbage tablets recently offered by a Dutch pharmaceutical firm.

What are these properties? There are almost too many to list. The Greek and Roman doctors of antiquity relied on cabbage as a universal panacea, using it indiscriminately both internally and externally, even against the plague.

Gradually over the centuries its specific qualities began to be sorted out. I imagine that cabbage has been the subject of more treatises and serious papers than any other vegetable. It has also been the most used of vegetables, even in modern times and in the teeth of public opinion. Many a distinguished doctor has not hesitated to bind a cabbage leaf over a particularly nasty wound, despite the risk of being called a quack. The results have always been remarkable.

The first time I myself used cabbage, I knew nothing about all this. I was just a young fellow and terribly in awe of my first patient, who happened to be one of the top men in the Vichy government. I was merely doing what my father, would have done, remembering how many times I had been sent out to the garden to find the best cabbage for him. So for my first consultation I had gone to the market square and come back with a cabbage, as well as a bunch of watercress and a fresh egg. With these purchases wrapped in a sheet of newspaper, I had presented myself at the great man's quarters. He was suffering from arthritis of the shoulder.

When I unwrapped my cabbage and asked for a vegetable chopper, I thought the great man was going to have me thrown out. Then his expression softened. I read in his face the humility of a man in physical pain. Despite his skepticism, he let me go on with my preparations. In my professional life I have always depended on this initial passive acceptance on the part of patients who are in actual pain. Otherwise, in their vanity, they would send me packing when they saw me unpacking my medicines. Thus I gain some time in which to demonstrate that my unlikely-looking plants have some surprising powers.

On that day my cabbage performed a miracle. I am still grateful to it. If it had failed me, that one time, I might perhaps have abandoned the profession I love so much. But the cabbage did not fail. I later learned the reasons why.

Captain Cook undertook a three-year sea voyage without losing a single man in his crew—an extraordinary thing in the eighteenth century. He is reported to have carried a cargo of cabbage in his hold. Cook must have been aware of the antiscorbutic properties of cabbage, as well as of its other medicinal uses. For in those days scurvy was a mysterious and dreaded disease claiming the lives of many sailors.

Since my own first successful experiment, I have read many studies on cabbage and know why it deserves its title of "the poor man's medicine."

In the first place, cabbage makes ideal first-aid material. Medicines are not always around in emergencies, but there might well be a cabbage in the garden, or at the nearest grocer's, which will serve splendidly both for bandage and antiseptic.

In case of a burn or an insect bite, a crushed cabbage leaf promptly applied relieves the pain and speeds the healing. Crushed cabbage is also good for any cut or sore, for lesions, pimples, abcesses, boils, etc.

Cabbage has the faculty of drawing out infection and suppuration from the skin. The wound should be washed with boiled water and a dressing of crushed cabbage applied. This should be renewed daily until complete healing has taken place.

For more serious wounds, the cabbage leaves should be plunged into boiling water for a few moments to soften them and make them more malleable. I often follow a procedure that my patients find amusing. I ask for an electric iron, and after cutting out the central rib, I iron my cabbage leaves until they are as soft as velvet. Even people in severe pain will smile at this trick. Another procedure is to soak the cabbage leaf in olive oil for an hour. The oil softens it, makes it cling better and increases its antiseptic effect.

In the days before sterilized gauze bandages were readily available, cabbage leaves were often used to bind up wounds. Even today, certain types of injuries, varicose veins, ulcerations, swelling, skin eruptions, hemorrhoids and superficial infections respond remarkably well to applications of cabbage.

The various muscular aches and pains, sciatica, neuralgia and rheumatism, are much relieved by hot compresses of cabbage, well chopped, wrapped in muslin and applied to the painful areas. My grandmother, who suffered from arthritis, used to tuck a cabbage leaf into her woollen knee guards. Many times I have seen old people in my part of the country slip a cabbage leaf into the flannel bindings with which they wrap their hips in wintertime.

I also recommend a hot compress of cabbage upon any painful area of the body. Used this way, cabbage relieves liver attacks, and placed over the stomach, is helpful against intestinal pains, diarrhea, dysentery and dysmenorrhea. Applied to the brow, it will sooth migraine. For colds and asthma, lay the hot compresses on chest and throat.

In cases of sore throat I recommend gargling with cabbage

juice (obtained easily with a juicer). For loss of voice, mix a few spoonfuls of honey with cabbage juice and drink it slowly.

Cabbage is enormously valuable when taken internally. I recommend it for cirrhosis of the liver, especially that caused by alcoholism, for dysentery, for all intestinal diseases. It is beneficial against anemia, arthritis and gout.

There is every good reason, then, to include cabbage in your diet. Use it in all its forms—as a juice, minced up raw in salads, in soups and stews. Stuffed cabbage makes a delicious main dish, and choucroute likewise, though you should avoid adding too much fatty sausage to this healthful vegetable.

I have found that cabbage water, brewed with a bit of sage, makes a soothing evening drink for people who tend to have nightmares.

From a nourishing morning broth suitable for the farmer leaving for his fields to an evening tea for the city man suffering from nervous strain, cabbage will serve you well all the day long. It is a lifelong guardian of health and a healer of wounds.

Carrot

You might think we hardly have to sing its praises, since the carrot occupies a privileged place among the garden vegetables. As everyone knows, carrots are good for the disposition. True enough. A person in excellent health will have a disposition to match.

It is also common knowledge that a dish of carrots will relieve a liver attack. And carrots are also prized as a beauty aid. Bright-colored themselves, they bring color to girls' cheeks.

Yet children often complain: Carrots again! And they have a valid point, for they have been eating carrots since the cradle. Strained carrots are usually the baby's first solid food. They are also a prime remedy for infants' digestive disorders. If your baby has diarrhea, dash out to the garden, pick a few carrots, stew them in a little water and put them through a mixer or a food mill. Feed him this purée instead of milk for a few days. When the diarrhea disappears, resume the milk again, but in half the usual quantity. The other half should be the carrot purée.

In country districts a baby's first toy will often be a raw peeled carrot. The child will cut its teeth on it: it tastes good, its firm texture is welcome and its orange color is pleasing to the baby's still dim vision.

As the child gets older, carrots should continue in his diet, for they are important to the growth process, strengthening the bones and preventing anemia. Their vitamin and mineral contents are extremely high. During World War II a carrot meal was developed to replace all the missing nutritional elements. It seems to have been most effective, even for keeping nursing mothers in milk.

But let us not reserve carrots for children or for emergency situations. They belong on the family table in all their forms— as carrot sticks, grated, in soups and stews, or boiled and lightly sautéed in butter. They can also be turned into a delicious juice. I am strongly in favor of all the vegetable juices, to be drunk at the start of a meal or first thing in the morning. Carrot juice, spiked with a sliver of lemon, is one of the tastiest.

Carrots should not be peeled, for their thin epidermis is rich in vitamins, while their heart contains little of these. I remember how my mother used to scrub carrots with a stiff brush and rinse them in cold water. That was all that was necessary. If your carrots come from your own garden and are grown without chemical fertilizer, you need not worry about them. If you do not know their origins, you will want to wash them somewhat more carefully.

Do not discard your carrot tops. They add a wonderful flavor to vegetable soups and are rich in minerals.

There are a host of external uses for carrots. Though somewhat less potent than cabbage, grated carrots may be made into poultices for cuts, burns and sores. An antiseptic decoction useful for sore throats and as a general mouthwash may be made from carrot tops.

I use carrots for many of my creams and beauty preparations (see Chapter 6). My father, to whom I am indebted for many of my recipes, used to handle carrots with the same tender care he gave to flowers. Since the carrot benefits delicate skins, he reasoned, it must itself be delicate.

One of the loveliest flowers of the fields and roadside is the wild carrot or Queen Anne's lace. It is a graceful plant, with its fine-cut foliage and white lacy flower head. Both its root, woodier and thinner than the cultivated carrot, and its seeds furnish excellent diuretic teas. Slice the root into small sections, gather the seeds and dry them for later use. Everything about the carrot is beneficent.

Celery

Did woman know what celery
Bestows upon a man,
She would go forth to search for it
From Rome to Turkestan.

Odd bits of doggerel like this are fun to collect. Almost always they will have a companion verse. In this case we find:

Did man but know what celery would do for him,
Nought else would fill his garden rim to rim.

What special property were these old jingles hinting at? The implication is that celery is an aphrodisiac and stimulates the sexual glands. Legend also has it that celery was an ingredient of the love potion that had such dire effects on Tristan and Isolde. To be sure, a number of esoteric elements went into that mixture—the testicles of a two-year-old white rooster, the flower of that strange herb, mandrake, and, in a more culinary vein, truffles, crayfish, pimento, pepper, cumin, thyme and bay leaf, all in wine. With company like this, who can say what part the simple garden vegetable had in inducing that fatal passion?

Celery has many other qualities to commend it. It is especially useful for people who want to slim down. I always tell my figure-conscious lady patients to eat a few stalks of celery between mealtimes. This appeases the appetite and helps maintain regularity. The cellulose in raw celery is excellent roughage.

Because of its depurative qualities, it is useful against diabetes, gout and rheumatism. For all these illnesses I recommend celery juice, perhaps mixed with carrot or tomato juice for a more interesting taste. During a rheumatic attack a glass of pure celery juice every day will do miracles. In Japan they treat rheumatism with complete celery cures. For a whole month patients are fed nothing but celery, in a variety of forms.

Lastly, celery has a calming effect on the nerves. This has

been known since antiquity, on no less an authority than Hippocrates. Today scientific research has established that celery is an excellent tonic for the nervous system. I prescribe it in cases of neurasthenia.

Celery root has the same virtues as stalk celery. It, too, may be eaten either raw or cooked. Celery tops may be easily dried, in the manner of other herbs, while the root may be cut in thin slices and likewise dried. Even though this vegetable is usually available in the market all year round, it is convenient to have it on hand in dried form. A handful of dried celery leaves contributes distinctive flavor to any sort of soup.

Watercress

The kitchen garden is no place for it. In thrives in sandy wet ground, preferably on the margin of a brook. Despite its remarkable virtues, many people shy away from it, for it has the reputation of causing liver fluke. Wild watercress may, in fact, harbor the worm that carries this serious disease. The leaves should therefore be soaked in salted water for an hour or two, or made into a soup.

Cultivated watercress is free of this danger and may and should be eaten freely, for it is exceptionally rich in vitamins, above all in vitamin C. It is also an excellent source of minerals, containing more iron than spinach, but no oxalic acid, which some people cannot tolerate. With its abundant content of oligo elements and iodine, it is a fine depurative.

I recommend it for the circulation, the liver and the skin. Since watercress stimulates the appetite, it also combats anemia.

A glass of watercress juice drunk upon waking in the morning has a bracing effect on the whole organism. If you find the taste somewhat strong, you may mix it with other vegetable juices. With the addition of onion juice, it wonderfully brightens and freshens the complexion.

Watercress also helps clear the lungs and relieves catarrh and congestion of the bronchi. I recommend watercress, coarsely chopped and added to a cup of bouillon, for tonsillitis.

In the past watercress salad would be prescribed for spells of dizziness. It is reputed to have been highly effective in restoring the sense of equilibrium.

I have found watercress a useful medicine for external infections. As I mentioned in the section on cabbage, I included watercress in my poultice against rheumatism. Patients with gout and rheumatism must be especially grateful for this vegetable, which benefits them either as a salad, a juice or a soup, and soothes their pain when applied externally.

Watercress is kind to the skin. Crushed and applied with a wad of cotton, it relieves irritations and helps heal acne and other skin conditions. It will also bleach out freckles, should anyone still consider them undesirable.

Perhaps this could be stated as a rule:

> *If you wish to have a lily-white skin*
> *Steep yourself in green without and within.*

Lettuce

We now come to the subject of salads, concerning which there are two schools of thought. Some believe in the overwhelming value of the green leafy vegetables, while others have nothing but contempt for them. "We are not cows," they say and insist upon more solid nourishment.

The truth lies somewhere in between. In sheer quantity, the value of greens may be a snare and a delusion. A child fed only salads would not form healthy bones. Persons with a tendency to edema or retention of fluids should eat the salad vegetables only in moderation. However, with these exceptions salad vegetables, especially lettuce, are rich in blessing.

Since they are eaten raw, the salad vegetables require careful handling. Where sanitary conditions are primitive, they may transmit typhoid, hepatitis or amebic dysentery. But these cases are extremely rare and should not be allowed to frighten us, especially since such dangers can be avoided. Always remember to wash your salad vegetables thoroughly, unless they come out of your own garden. Drop a bit of permanganate into the water, or let them soak for an hour in water with some lemon juice or vinegar.

Lettuce has long been called "the herb of wisdom." We may wonder why. Does browsing make us wise? Possibly it does. But lettuce has earned its name more by virtue of its calming qualities, its sedative, even hypnotic effect.

Trusting in this principle, I undertook to treat an American millionairess who had long been suffering from insomnia. She had tried all sorts of cures in vain. When she came to me, her nerves were at the breaking point. I advised her to eat three braised lettuces every evening for dinner. Why braised, she asked. Because they were less discouraging that way, I answered. After all, three fresh lettuces would fill a monster salad bowl. However, if she preferred them raw, they would do her just as much good.

My patient departed for home with a good many packets of French lettuce seed in her luggage. Because, she explained, such varieties were unknown in the United States. She had the lettuce planted in her country estate and applied herself to her lettuce cure. For fifteen years now she has regularly sent me a Christmas card with the note: "I sleep, I sleep." Moreover she has spread the gospel among her neighbors and friends, who now also grow a little patch of lettuce. So there is one corner of the United States where sleeping pills are unnecessary.

Lettuce is at its medicinal best when it has bolted to seed. It then contains a milky juice whose sedative, narcotic and even anesthetic qualities have been well recognized by the pharmaceutical houses. From this syrup they have compounded a host of products prescribed for nervous disorders, whooping cough, menstrual pain, intestinal spasm and similar troubles.

Along with lettuce's powers to cure insomnia and nightmares, it can also allay excessive physical desire. An old name for it is "the herb of eunuchs." This may not be so at odds with its other name—"The herb of wisdom"—for continence and wisdom surely have points in common. At any rate, one can confidently prescribe lettuce to decrease sexual excitement.

Nevertheless, people should not avoid eating lettuce on this account. In one of those paradoxes dear to nature, lettuce is also the plant of fertility. Lettuce is exceptionally rich in vitamin E, a key element in the reproductive process, for it is essential to the maturation of the ovum. What a remarkable vegetable, which both helps us sleep and helps women bear fine children!

Cucumber

With our wealth of vegetables, we tend to rate the cucumber rather low. The general opinion is that it is almost all water and has little flavor. Yet cucumbers are held in high esteem in Eastern Europe, which lacks the abundance and variety of green vegetables we revel in.

In these parts of the world cucumbers are preserved in brine and kept in barrels for the winter months. The liquid they give off is saved and used in cooking. Hence it grieves me when I see the housewife prepare a salad from sliced cucumbers from which she has first pressed all the liquid. It is as though she had squeezed oranges and thrown away the juice. What is more, I would advise against peeling the cucumber, for its green skin is rich in vitamins.

The first and foremost use of cucumbers is as a diuretic. As such it helps cleanse the body of its toxins and can do great things for the figure. It is excellent practice to eat a good dish of cucumbers every evening. Slice them but do not peel them, season them with garlic and parsley, olive oil and lemon juice and watch yourself grow slimmer. Women troubled by cellulite will find their spongy tissues firm up wonderfully, for cucumber dissolves uric acid and superfluous fat.

Cucumbers are also delicious cooked and should perhaps be eaten so by people with delicate digestions. Slice the cucumbers and simmer them in a little water, or put them through a food mill or a mixer to form a purée for a soup. A few slices of fresh cucumber makes a good addition to any vegetable juice.

Nowadays we are all aware of the virtues of cucumber for external use. Many cosmetic firms use cucumbers in their masks and beauty creams. I, too, use cucumber for this purpose. Nor is there any need to buy expensive preparations, for you can make your own beauty lotions from the cucumbers in your garden. These will have the further advantage of being fresh and free of chemical additives.

When you are preparing a cucumber salad for guests, do not throw away the liquid you have pressed from your cucumbers. While you are busy in the kitchen, apply the liquid to your face with a wad of cotton. When your company arrives they will be astonished to find the cook looking so dewy and fresh in spite of her labors over the hot stove.

You will also find cucumber juice or cucumber slices a soothing treatment for burns and sunburn.

Artichoke

You probably eat only its heart. But I use every part of the plant—flower, stem, leaves and root. When you have come to appreciate this great and lordly denizen of the kitchen garden, you, too, will want to make the most of it.

Perhaps you trim away the outer petals of baby artichokes and serve them raw, sprinkled with salt. The larger ones you boil. But do not discard the water in which you have cooked your artichokes, for it is rich in mineral salts and adds subtle flavor to soups and stews.

Most people know that artichokes are beneficial to the liver. Anyone suffering from a liver complaint will feel much better after an artichoke cure. But artichoke also offers good protection against urea, cholesterol, intestinal viruses and arthritis. It is both diuretic and depurative.

So be brave and follow me into the garden. We will fell a stout artichoke plant with a sickle, cut up its stem, strip off its leathery leaves, pull up its root and carry our booty to the kitchen. But this is not where bravery is required. The real test of your courage comes in drinking the potions we are going to prepare from the plant. We may press out the juices of the stem and leaves. We may steep the root in white wine. But whatever we do, be prepared for a bitter taste. Camomile is the mildest of beverages compared to this.

Nevertheless, once you have gotten used to it, you may even find the flavor enjoyable. Two or three spoonfuls taken before meals, perhaps in a glass of madeira, will keep rheumatism away from you your whole life. A tisane brewed from the fresh leaves is excellent medication for a liver attack. You may make a face while you down your dose of artichoke. But remember that you are being spared the agonies of a liver attack or the pangs of rheumatism.

If you simply do not have it in you to be a hero, there are artichoke preparations you can buy at the pharmacist's which have been treated in certain ways to counteract the bitterness.

Tomato

The tomato is a comparative newcomer to Europe. Brought from Peru by the Spanish conquistadors, it was first grown as an ornamental plant under the flattering name of love-apple. The very seductiveness of its appearance made it suspect as an edible fruit. Now, of course, we know that it is as good as it looks, though there are still some people who shy away from the tomato because of its acidity. For those who must exercise this kind of care, tomatoes are better eaten raw than cooked.

Yet it is precisely the acidity of the tomato, along with its high content of vitamins and minerals, that makes it an effective agent against stomach acidity, constipation, viscosity of the blood, uremia, kidney and bladder stones, gout and arthritis.

I would urge people with a tendency toward gout and rheumatism to drink a large glass of freshly pressed tomato juice every day throughout the summer. For a refinement of flavor, add a bit of celery juice to the potion.

The special fragrance of the tomato leaves, like mild cinnamon, is pleasing to our senses but apparently not so to insects. Thus your row of tomato plants out in the kitchen garden is protecting all the other vegetables from bugs and worms. If you hang a bouquet of dried tomato leaves in all the rooms of your house, you will not be troubled by flies, mosquitoes or spiders. In my part of France people have long depended on this method. This is a far healthier way to banish insects than by heavily spraying your house with insect bombs.

Tomato leaves are also effective antidotes to the poison of insect bites. Should you be stung by a bee or a wasp, run to the garden, and rub the affected spot with tomato leaves.

Spinach

By now no one needs to be told how healthful spinach is. Its special merit lies in its high iron content, which affects the blood and the muscles. Spinach is also rich in chlorophyll, vitamins and sundry minerals. I recommend spinach especially to people with anemia, to growing children, to convalescents and to anyone with a liver or stomach complaint.

Though we usually eat it boiled, in a variety of tempting dishes, we might also try it raw as an interesting addition to a salad. Put through a juicer, spinach yields an excellent drink. Mixed with the juice of watercress, it will truly be an elixir of health.

A word of warning: I would absolutely forbid spinach to people with gout or rheumatism. It contains oxalic acid, which is dangerous for them. Knowledge of vegetables consists in recognizing such fine points, for a generally beneficial nutrient may be a bane to someone with a specific health problem. The principal thing is to be conscious of what you are eating and adjust your diet to your individual needs.

Chicory

Hardly anyone would single out the wild chicory as a beautiful plant. Yet it is the first to open its flowers at break of day. Many a time I have encountered its ragged blue bloom at five in the morning, when I set out to gather herbs with the dew still on them, and have admired the way the pale and fragile petals of the chicory match the mists lifting from the fields. I greet it respectfully and to me it is a lovely plant for I know its powers. As with women, the more humble plants are often the richest in hidden goodness.

Every part of the wild chicory is beneficial—its leaves, its roots. Of course we are better acquainted with its cultivated descendants—curly escarole, the crisp sprouts of endive and the heavy-headed, somewhat rumpled Batavian chicory whose blanched yellow heart makes so refreshing a salad. All these enhance our table and contribute to our health, but not to the same degree as the wild plant. As always, the wild plant is more tonic.

Too often in preparing a salad we throw away the large outer leaves of our head of chicory. This is a great mistake from both the nutritional and the gastronomic viewpoint. Keep these leaves, simmer them a moment or two in water and you will have the tenderest and tastiest of greens. They are wonderful for regulating the liver and the flow of bile. People with jaundice should eat quantities of chicory.

Wild chicory is especially helpful for diabetes. It can be taken either in the form of a tea or a juice, perhaps mixed with the juice of watercress. For people of normal health, chicory acts as a tonic, a diuretic, a depurative and a mild laxative.

Then there is roasted and ground chicory root, which in former days would often serve as a breakfast beverage in many families. Even today the thrifty housewife can stretch her coffee beans by mixing them with a few spoonfuls of chicory. The resulting drink is particularly good for children and people with liver problems. Certain brands of instant coffee include chicory to accentuate the coffee's flavor. But some of the chicory's virtues are certainly lost in the processing. My advice would be to revive the habit of drinking chicory by itself. It makes a delicious hearty beverage for the whole family and is far easier to digest than coffee.

Dandelion

I hardly know whether to classify the dandelion as an herb or a vegetable. While essentially a wild plant, it is well known and appreciated as an addition to our table, particularly in early spring. A dish of tender young dandelion leaves dressed with oil, vinegar and bits of fried bacon is an epicure's delight. So while the dandelion is equally prized by the pharmacists, let us call it a vegetable.

As with chicory, every part of the dandelion has its uses. Wild animals seek it out and doctor themselves on its leaves. Domesticated rabbits are mad about dandelion, and will devour as much of it as they are given. In the spring country women go out in the fields, armed with basket and knife, to hunt down the rosettes of early dandelion. Such a hunt is hard on the back, but the women know that what they bring home is well worth the hours of stooping.

Dandelion is a superlative diuretic, as its name in French (*pissenlit*) indicates. It is a boon to the difficult liver. It is equally beneficial in cases of diabetes, cellulite, skin troubles, gout and rheumatism.

While the leaves of dandelion are used for salad and greens, its root yields a fine tisane when simmered a while in a quantity of water. A juice may also be pressed from its roots and a teaspoonful of this, several times a day, will be good for almost anything that ails you. We have an expression in France about eating the dandelion by its roots. It means much the same as the English expression "pushing up the daisies." But I contend that it is much better to eat the dandelion root while one is still aboveground.

Dandelion root may be treated in much the same way as chicory root. Dig it up in the autumn when it has attained a fair size, cut it into slices, roast it and grind it to make a comforting warm drink. Like chicory, it is tonic, laxative and diuretic.

The white sap that trickles out of a broken dandelion stalk is a potent medicine. It will make warts disappear. It is also used as an eyewash: one drop in each eye dispels infection.

Only the white silk of the ripened blossom goes to waste. But since each bit of flying fluff carries a seed, we must grant that it, too, is highly functional.

Radish

We are all familiar with the small scarlet buttons that add crispness and piquancy to salads and open sandwiches. But there are also the large white radishes, which mature later in the summer and can be grated for a refreshing salad or nibbled along with a glass of beer. Then there are the black radishes, which are harvested last of all and can be stored for winter keeping. In Germany, Hungary, Poland and Russia this variety is much prized. There is also the horseradish, a perennial plant closely related to the wild radish. Its biting sharpness has earned it the country name of capuchin mustard. We need dig up only a few inches of its long root, grate it and mix it with vinegar for a condiment.

All have in common a piquant taste that increases salivation and whets the appetite. I recommend radishes for sickly children and people with anemia. Serve a plateful of little radishes as an hors d'oeuvre. Put older radishes that have grown large and knobby through a juicer, cutting the resulting liquid with carrot juice if you find it too sharp. Sprinkle radish slices on top of a cold soup. In any guise the radish is valuable.

Nevertheless, I would advise people with delicate digestions to observe moderation in eating radishes. Strong radishes can give such a shock to the lining of the stomach as to cause vomiting. While in small quantities the radish stimulates the lazy stomach, in larger doses it produces violent contractions. The mucous tissues of the throat and lungs are especially susceptible to the sting of radish. Hence it can be very useful against respiratory infections. You will find a host of cough syrups at the pharmacist's which have radish for their base. In Siberia, where pharmacists are few and far between, the natives concoct a simple syrup that is especially good against bronchitis. It consists of one part juice of radish to two parts honey. A tablespoon of this mixture before every meal and at bedtime soon clears away the phlegm and relieves a sore throat.

Some forms of stubborn asthma can be relieved by a homemade horseradish preparation. Make it up in small amounts, since it is better when fresh. Grate a piece of horseradish as fine as possible, mix it with lemon juice and take this by the teaspoonful several times a day, between meals. More than this you will hardly be able to stand. It will bring tears to your eyes but the burning sensation as it goes down your throat is proof of its potency. By and by you will become hardened to it.

This medicine is not for you if you have a delicate stomach or are afflicted by hemorrhoids or other inflammations. The stinging action of radish will exacerbate these troubles.

I give the opposite advice to people with arthritis and rheumatism. They can freely use radish as a poultice. Applied to the painful spots of the body, it produces a pleasant tingle and dispels the ache.

Another recommendation: A bit of horseradish, chewed slowly, will help to harden the gums and prevent abcesses and loosening of the teeth.

There is an old wives' recipe concerning radish which I have never tested but which does not seem devoid of logic, so I will offer it here: In case of insomnia, nightmares or troubled sleep, smear each of your calves with a layer of grated radish. This will draw the blood from your congested brain to your legs. Slumber is supposed to follow soon after. The treatment may well work.

In any case, remember that radishes are dynamite, to be used with caution. But their power for good is also formidable .

Fennel

Fennel has long been the subject of ribald jokes—in Rabelais, for instance. The reason is that fennel is famous for its "carminative" properties—that is, it causes the expelling of intestinal wind. But this is certainly to the plant's honor. Hence the old custom of cooking some wisps of wild fennel along with other vegetables that are difficult to digest, like beans and cabbage, makes perfect sense. The fennel stimulates the contractions of the intestines.

Nowadays, I am glad to say, the sweet fennel so appreciated in Italy has become a common vegetable in our markets, and not only in the south of France where it originated. It is easily raised in any soil, provided the climate is suitable, for it does require a longish growing season. It surely belongs in the home garden, and on your table.

You can eat it raw as an hors' d'oeuvre, or separate its stalks and serve them as you would celery. Mix its juice with that of other fresh vegetables, or include it in your salads where its delicate anise flavor complements that of all the other ingredients. It is splendid in soups and makes a delicious dish baked with oil and dusted with grated cheese.

In all these forms it has the merit of being easily digested, soothing to the stomach and the intestines, mildly laxative and diuretic.

What is more, fennel has the faculty of regularizing menstrual periods and normalizing an insufficient flow. Hence its reputation as an abortifacient, when in fact it merely has a relaxing effect on the reproductive organs. In the past parsley was also classified as an abortifacient, for the same reasons. I find such an interpretation all too mechanical. In fact, from the medical standpoint, any plant that stimulates menstruation is favorable to conception, insofar as it restores the woman to full health.

I therefore recommend fennel without any reservations whatever. It even increases the milk supply of nursing mothers.

Like lettuce, then, fennel is rich in benefactions for the family. Perhaps it should be made an emblem of happy domestic life.

Asparagus

Here is a vegetable greatly esteemed by gourmets and served at the very best tables. But even apart from its interesting taste, asparagus has a function to perform in the course of a meal: eaten at the beginning, it stimulates the appetite; eaten toward the end, it acts as a laxative and digestive.

Asparagus is beneficial for a lazy liver and for diabetes. Its tonic properties make it an appropriate food for intellectuals for it heightens the mental and emotional faculties. Yet for this very reason people suffering from insomnia or overwrought nerves should keep away from asparagus. Let them have a good salad instead.

Curiously enough, the same vegetable that is excitant to the brain and nerves has a calming effect on heart ailments and palpitations. Again paradoxically, while asparagus is highly recommended for rheumatism because it promotes elimination, it is forbidden in cases of rheumatic fever. Similarly, it is dangerous for people with urinary problems, prostate trouble or gonorrhea.

Thus asparagus is a vegetable of double aspect and should be treated with care.

Turnip and Rutabaga

Unfortunately, these two vegetables have bad associations, for they are linked in our minds with wartime and general scarcity and so have come to symbolize privation. Moreover, we have made the word "turnip" pejorative, saying that something or other is not worth a turnip, or that a dull person is a turniphead. Thus turnips have been cast into disrepute.

This is a pity, for turnips have much to commend them. Do not omit turnips from your garden or from your soups, for a turnip or two, diced small or puréed, adds a subtle flavor to the whole which will make your guests exclaim: "There is something special in this soup." I hope you have character enough to confess what it is and thus help rehabilitate the good turnip.

Young turnips boiled, then lightly browned in the juices of a roast duck, satisfy the most exacting gourmet. Glazed, they make a splendid accompaniment to pork, beef or fowl.

Make generous use of turnip, for like its large cousin, the rutabaga, it is rich in minerals, vitamins and fruit sugars. It is good for children, for people with anemia, for people on a reducing diet and for those with bronchitis, tonsillitis or gout.

A good medicine for chest colds can be made from it. Boil the turnip until soft, put it through a food mill and mix the pulp with milk to which a few spoonfuls of honey have been added. The resulting drink is pleasant, curative and nutritious. An effective gargle can be made from the water in which the turnip was boiled.

Just as turnip is helpful in soothing the sore throat caused by tonsillitis, it is an excellent treatment for chilblains, chapped skin or boils. Bake the turnip, mash it and apply directly to the affected areas.

Rhubarb

Our grandmothers used to make wonderful sauces, pies and preserves from its rosy stems. It satisfied our hunger for fruit in the early spring before any other fruit was remotely ready. Nowadays rhubarb seems to have become almost a rarity in the market. So put in a few roots of rhubarb at the end of your garden. They will supply you with all you can use, spring after spring, while the plants themselves make a stately garden accent all summer long, their wrinkled dark green leaves recalling the Himalayas from which the plant originally came.

Rhubarb yields a strong purgative which should be used with care. I have heard that nursing mothers who have eaten rhubarb transmit this purgative action in their milk to their babies. On the other hand, a simple dish of stewed rhubarb will put an end to an attack of bilious diarrhea. If this is a chronic condition, rhubarb will eliminate the causes of the trouble.

The pharmacist offers a host of preparations based on rhubarb root. But the fresh plant is a source of continuous health.

Strawberry and Raspberry

A bed of strawberries belongs in every kitchen garden. The plants are of easy culture and with proper management will provide a rich harvest of berries for years on end.

Who does not love strawberries? But how many are aware of the dainty berry's high vitamin content, or its quotient of precious iron? Hence it is especially recommended for people with anemia, for convalescents and for the aged.

What is more, strawberries are a prime depurative. If some people find that eating strawberries makes them break out in a rash, this is usually because the disintoxication produced by the strawberries is so rapid that the poisons simply rise to the skin, creating the blotches. These subside after a little while and are nothing to worry about. They by no means signify a real allergy.

Because of its depurative properties, the strawberry is recommended for sufferers from arthritis and rheumatism as well as for those with liver complaints. For maximum benefit, strawberries should be eaten at the beginning of a meal rather than at the end. Better still would be to wake early, take a stroll in the garden and eat the berries that have ripened overnight. On the other hand, if you want a good diuretic, do without your regular supper and eat a quart of strawberries instead. Go to bed early and in the morning you will empty your bladder with a rare feeling of well-being, for your entire system will have been cleansed. In addition, you will have passed a remarkably restful night, for strawberries contain a bromide that promotes sleep.

A strawberry cure of several days' duration will bring great relief to people with gout or kidney stones.

A few drops of vinegar on your sugared strawberries makes them easier to digest, besides intensifying their flavor. Lemon juice will do the same.

Strawberries are among those rare fruits permitted to diabetics, since their particular form of sugar, levulose, is easily assimilated. Strawberries can also be enjoyed as a thirst-quencher, if eaten without sugar.

Strawberry leaves have a lovely delicate flavor and may be picked, dried and kept for winter use. Country people use the leaves for tea. The leaves may also be brewed into medicinal diuretics and depuratives.

Even the root of the strawberry plant is useful. Gathered and dried in the springtime or fall, the root will yield decoctions effective against diarrhea and gout. Do not be alarmed if your urine has a reddish tint after drinking this tea—that is a normal effect of the strawberry root and implies nothing wrong.

Women have long known that they can make their faces sparkle by rubbing their skin with slices of ripe strawberry. The moisture of the fruit passes instantly into the pores and the tired skin is revitalized.

Raspberries have the same diuretic and tonic qualities as strawberries. Diabetics may regale themselves on raspberries. They are also good for rheumatism. Dried raspberry leaves make pleasant tea with a mildly laxative action. For a heavenly dessert, mix strawberries and raspberries in a fruit salad. You will not only be eating wonderfully but doing yourself the utmost good.

Currant and Gooseberry

Alongside of your strawberry bed, why not have a neat hedge of red and black currants? It will not only trim your garden beautifully, but it will also yield a cupboardful of jams and jellies.

If you can have only one fruit in your garden, it should be the currant, the richest of all fruits in vitamin C. Moreover, its C content is especially stable and does not suffer in processing. The various syrups, wines, liqueurs and preserves made from currants may all be considered elixirs of life. The city of Dijon enjoys a certain fame as the center of the currant liqueur industry. But every housewife used to treasure her family recipes for currant syrups and preserves, and would put up many jars of these in years when the harvest was generous and the price of the fruit reasonable.

So drink your fill of these delicious beverages, remembering that they also counter fatigue and fend off liver ailments and arthritis. Fresh currant juice or currant syrup is also useful for combating colds or throat infections. Dried currant leaves make a diuretic tea that is effective against rheumatism and bladder problems. The leaves should be picked before or after the bush has flowered, that is to say, in April or August, when you will not interfere with its fruiting.

The small jagtoothed currant leaves, with their characteristic pleasant perfume, are also good against insect bites. You have only to rub a few leaves over the bite and it will stop hurting.

Gooseberries have the same qualities as currants but to a somewhat lesser degree.

A favorite preserve of the old days was the so-called four-fruit mixture, made up of strawberries, raspberries, currants and gooseberries, sometimes with cherries thrown in for good measure.

Blackberry

You will have to step out of your garden to find them, but you will probably not have far to go. Ask your children and they will lead you to the hedgerow where they have been happily feasting on the glistening jet-black fruits.

Pick a quart for immediate eating with sugar and cream, and another for jellies and juices. These are even more welcome in the winter than in the summertime, especially since blackberry syrup helps fend off tonsillitis and chest colds.

Although the ripe berry is a laxative, the green berry has the opposite effect and may be used to combat diarrhea, especially in small infants. A few spoonfuls of syrup made from the unripe berries will settle their bowels promptly.

As for the leaves of the blackberry canes, I treasure them even more than I do the fruit in which I gloried through all the summers of my youth. I make a practice of gathering the young shoots in spring, soon after the leaves unfurl. Dried, they lend themselves to a variety of uses. They can be brewed into tisanes for curbing diarrhea and dysentery. Made into a gargle, they clear up throat infections and heal any lesion of the gums.

Infusions of blackberry leaves also make an excellent douching mixture for women troubled by leukhorrea.

Blueberry

If you go to the mountains for your vacation, you will enjoy taking your family out to pick blueberries, or as we call them in France "grapes of the woodland."

Blueberries are wonderful with sugar and cream or made into muffins and fritters. They are equally precious converted into jams and jellies, juices or liqueurs. Medically, they are useful against diarrhea, especially in children, dysentery and any intestinal upset. Laboratory experiments have established that blueberry juice can destroy certain dangerous microbes. This would explain the traditional practice of prescribing blueberry syrup for stubborn intestinal ailments.

Blueberries can improve sluggish circulation. Interestingly enough, they also benefit eyesight, particularly nocturnal vision. Hence blueberries are recommended fare for airplane pilots who need eagle-sharp eyes to see through the clouds. Young air force officers are always pleased to be served blueberry tarts at mess, but they usually do not know the reason why. People who do considerable night driving should also include a generous share of blueberries in their diet.

Blueberries have a healing effect on any infection of the mouth. The fresh berries may either be mashed and applied to the blistered area, or boiled in a pint of water and used as a gargle. A similar solution makes a soothing lotion for hemorrhoids.

A medicinal tea for the control of diabetes may be made from the leaves.

Apple

Let us return to your garden. If you could plant but a single tree, it should be an apple tree.

The health-giving properties of the apple have always been appreciated. Remember that old saying: An apple a day keeps the doctor away.

If an apple comes from your own garden, you may eat it skin and all. But if it has been raised commercially, you had better peel it. Unfortunately, this is true for all the fruits whose skins were once savory and healthful but which nowadays are so saturated with chemicals that they have become dangerous.

The uses of apples are almost too many to name. Grated fine, apple is a favorite with babies. Stew apples for sauce, or for a richer taste, sauté them in a little butter and sprinkle with brown sugar and cinnamon. Simplest of all is to core them and pop them into the oven. Baked apples are delicious hot or cold.

Do not mistrust a misshapen apple—this is only a sign that it was grown without sprays. Some friends of mine who bought a place near Paris found that the apple trees in their orchard yielded a heavy crop. Though the quality was not up to commercial standards, the apples were remarkably tasty and free of worms. My friends wanted to give them to acquaintances, but people are so brainwashed by what they see in the stores that everybody hastily declined the gift. My friends offered their crop to a charitable organization and were again repulsed. And all because the apples had a mottled skin! What a mistake!

Sometimes in France a local army camp will take the excess crop when no one else will. The unit is in luck, for a bountiful supply of apples will keep the men in the best of health. An apple cure is good for everyone, men and women, young and old. It will bring tangible benefits to pregnant women and the overweight, to people with liver complaints and rheumatism, and even (to a certain degree) to diabetics. In addition, apples have a calming effect on the nerves and combat migraine and insomnia. Eat an apple at bedtime and you will enjoy a good night's sleep. Moreover, your teeth will be the whiter for it, and remain free of cavities, for apple disinfects the mouth.

If the apples come from your own garden, keep the cores and peelings for drying. They are even richer in benefits than the flesh of the fruit. Tisanes made of these parts are good for the heart and relieve the pangs of gout.

People in Normandy claim that their famous cider has the same virtues. However, we should drink cider moderately, for it has an acidifying effect. Since it is alcoholic, it should not be given to children.

Fresh apple juice makes a fine beauty lotion, cleansing the pores and firming the tissues.

In spring, when your apple tree is white with blossoms, gather a few handfuls of petals. Dried, these make a delicate infusion which is good against sore throats and coughs.

Cherry

The second fruit tree in your garden should be the cherry tree. You will then be able to make a springtime cure of fresh cherries: eat nothing else for two or three days running, and you will feel reborn, for the cherry is an excellent depurative. Diabetics may eat their fill of this fruit, for its sugar is highly assimilable. Cherries, low in calories, are highly recommended for people on a reducing diet. However, people with delicate intestines should eat them stewed.

The virtues of cherry stems are well known, for health food shops sell packages of stems for use as diuretic tea. Keep in mind that your own cherries are far better for this purpose because they have been grown without chemical sprays. Too often when we purchase natural products we expect will do us all kinds of good, we are instead inviting dangerous reactions because of their hidden content of chemicals and preservatives.

Peach, Apricot and Pear

I do not mean to deal with every single type of fruit available in the market or easily grown at home. They are all rich in vitamins and can serve as basis for a health and beauty cure. Eat them separately and mixed together in delicious fruit cocktails. A few pointers: The peach is diuretic and laxative; the apricot highly nutritious, rich in vitamin A, which is essential to growth and recommended for both the intellectual and the athlete. Pears are thirst-quenching, depurative and a rich source of minerals.

Of course, you are already aware of the virtues of the orange and all its relations (tangerines, lemons, grapefruit) as sources of vitamin C.

Plum

The third tree in your garden should be a plum tree. Perhaps saying this marks me as a chauvinist, but my part of France is famous for its plum trees and I can hardly do without this fruit.

The plum is a dynamic fruit, energy-giving and stimulating to the nerves. It is recommended for overworked executives and for athletes in training.

The juice of fresh plums is laxative, while the dried prune is even more so. A dish of stewed prunes for breakfast will prevent constipation and make any other measures unnecessary.

Thanks to a vigorous advertising campaign, plums are coming back into favor in France. For a while the fruit was almost in eclipse, but perhaps the arrival on the market of the dried California prune has spurred our own plum growers to a healthy rivalry. At any rate, we should all rejoice at the many recipes which have lately been appearing in the press, which greatly expand our ideas of how to use these delicious fruits. Try your hand at making plum preserves. Your family will be grateful in the winter months.

Gather and dry some plum leaves. These yield teas as diuretic and laxative as the fruit.

Grape

As a good Frenchman and a native of Gascony, where viticulture occupies an important place, I naturally assign a place of honor to the grape. But though I appreciate a good glass of wine, I am inclined to treat it prudently. I will have more to say on wine in Chapter 8. On the other hand, I cannot sufficiently praise the virtues of the fresh grape.

Autumn is the time for a radical grape cure, when the fruit is ripe and has stored up the summer's sun. Limit your diet to grapes for a week or two, consuming from two to four pounds per day. If you live in grape-growing country, this will be easier and more natural to carry out, but almost anywhere the price is down and the fruit is fresh. You will come out of your cure with a brand new liver, a cleansed digestive tract and in prime form to face the stresses of winter. The bicarbonate content of the grape is so high that it is superior to Vichy water as a disintoxicant.

Make sure you wash your grapes carefully to remove all traces of chemicals. However, the copper sulphate used for spraying grapes from time immemorial does not seem to have the injurious effect that the new chemicals have.

Since grapes are rich in natural sugars, you will not feel in the least hungry or weakened on a grape diet. There is a theory that grapes, like milk, constitute a complete food. They have even been compared to mother's milk.

In earlier years at harvest time people in the grape-growing districts would make a special preserve called *raisiné*. It is the most healthful preserve known. Recipes for it appear in Chapter 8, in the hope that people will rediscover this fine food.

Grapes, whether eaten plain or made into juice, are highly beneficial to children, pregnant women and athletes, all of whom expend unusual energy. Grapes are equally good for people with liver complaints, rheumatism or hypertension, as well as for people with skin diseases. Only diabetics should be warned against them, because of their high sugar content.

Dried raisins are high in energy and benefit the lungs. Give a handful to your children instead of candy and their health will thrive.

The adventurous cook might try using the juice of unripe grapes in place of lemon juice. You will appreciate the subtle difference in flavor. Or heap fresh grapes around your roast. They help draw out the fat and make the meat more digestible. The same might be done with goose liver *pâté*, cooked in the Gascon fashion. Garnished with grapes, this dangerously rich dish at once becomes more wholesome.

An oil rich in vitamin E is extracted from grape seeds. It is recommended for people with high cholesterol levels or with heart trouble. But gastronomes know still another use for grape seeds—certain creamy cheeses are rolled in grape seeds and absorb a distinctive flavor.

Grape leaves should be recognized as a first-rate green vegetable in their own right. To be sure, we know how they are used in Greek cookery, but we ought to use the tender pretty leaves more often as a green, like spinach.

The grape vine exhudes a sap after pruning—the so-called tears of the grape—which helps heal wounds and sores.

Only the black and gnarled grape stalks seem to have no use—except that they might make good walking sticks for oldsters who can ascribe their spryness to their lifelong devotion to the grape.

4. The Secrets of Herbs

I hope the foregoing little sketches will stand you and your family in good stead. Of course, you already knew something about the value of the various fruits and vegetables. However, in discussing herbs, I notice many people feel they have entered unknown territory—especially when I speak of their medicinal powers. Many people regard herbal medicine as a bizarre, outmoded science on a par with alchemy. And yet nothing is so simple as the "science of simples." Our ancestors profited from its secrets without having made any study of either botany or medicine. Certain time-honored procedures were known to have certain curative effects. That was all there was to it.

Therefore I beg you to put aside whatever biases you may have on this subject. We are simply setting out to discover what every housewife used to know in the days when she herself compounded healing teas, gargles and poultices to treat the minor illnesses of her family.

We are going to make the acquaintance of the good herbs. A number of them are happily at home in our kitchen gardens. These are the aromatic herbs used in cooking: parsley, tarragon, thyme, rosemary, sage, basil and savory. Others grow wild in the fields and along the roadsides: mints, mallow, poppy, plantain, horsetail, borage, celandine. Many have salty old names descriptive of their uses: fever herb, herb of the beaten woman, scurvy herb, tumbledown herb, centaur herb, donkey herb, corn herb, passion flower and so on. The list is very long.

My father, who knew no scientific nomenclature, called them by such names. For my part, I know them by several epithets, but I hardly ever find myself referring to them by their proper Latin designation. For they are old friends and the country names seem to suit them.

There are also the good herbs of the hedgerow (hawthorn, sloeberry), those growing on walls and ledges, those growing in cultivated fields (hops, Indian corn), those in the uplands (heather, gentians, ferns), or those in our pleasure gardens (rose, nasturium, marigold).

Teach your children to recognize them all. In the past children knew what the different flowers were called. Learning to identify plants can be a happy game. The children will range far and wide and come home with hands full of leaves and flowers. They will press their pickings between the pages of a heavy volume. In the evenings or on Sunday they and their parents can look up their specimens in a botanical manual and mount each flower on a separate sheet of paper, carefully writing its name underneath in their best penmanship. A small portfolio of this kind may become a child's precious possession. In any case, the child will not forget the names he has learned, or the happy hours of searching out these flowers.

My father had such a collection which he used to call his "herb notebook." It was supplemented with drawings, commentary and poems that he had written. Every so often we would look at it together and he would say: "See, my boy, this is my book of gold."

And I would be filled with reverence for all the wealth this book contained.

If you carry out this project along with your children, you will discover that it is not difficult to become a "master of plants." All it takes is a little application and considerable love. In a summer or two you can earn the degree. It is not one I reserve for myself, although the Post and Telegraph Service seems to think so, for I am sometimes forwarded letters from abroad addressed simply to Master of Plants, Paris, France.

If the day comes when there are millions of masters of plants about, the Post and Telegraph Service will have one more problem to cope with, but perhaps mankind will have fewer. I know a bit about the postal service, having been connected with the mail censorship department during the war. Many times I would hold a suspicious letter up to the light, shake it, sniff it, considering whether it should be checked or not. So I can easily imagine how refreshing it must be for present-day postal employees to smell some dried plant material through an envelope—a wisp of scorpion grass or a rose petal or perhaps the fragrance wafting from a package of mint or lavender sent by some kindly grandmother to her family in the city.

I myself am always sending such poetical little packages to friends to let them know they are in my thoughts. I also dispatch packets of my favorite herbs to various African heads of state who have come to me for medical advice and cannot obtain certain plants in their own country. Then, too, I exchange herbs with foreign plant healers, for we have much to learn from each other. Recently a professor from the faculty of the University of Colombia (they have always maintained a chair of herbal medicine at Bogotá) wrote to me proposing that we exchange some of our lore.

I think it a great pity that French universities have abolished their departments of herbal medicine, so that one can no longer earn a proper certificate in this field. Thus the profession of herbalist has disappeared, to the profit of the licensed pharmacist. It was the dream of my grandmother Sophie that I would someday rise to the status of pharmacist. My father's ambition was that I would become a government official, while my mother dreamed I would be a policeman. But I myself cannot imagine anything better than being an herbalist. I am never so happy as when I am home in my herb room in Gavarret, surrounded by the fragrant crocks of dried plants.

At the turn of the century the production of medicinal herbs in France started to fall sharply. There were fewer and fewer people who cared to make a living gathering herbs, and most of what we used was imported from abroad, from countries where labor was cheaper. During the First World War the government was quite worried about this, for medicinal herbs were badly needed, so measures were taken to encourage herb-gathering. These incentives worked so well that for a time there was even a surplus and France could export herbs. But during the 1920s the science of herbs fell gradually into oblivion. Nowadays the situation is even more deteriorated—with the encroachments of modern life into the country, and the creeping menace of pollution, good herbs are becoming scarcer and thus unprofitable to gather on a commercial basis.

My advice is that we all assure ourselves of our supply of herbs so that we do not need to depend so much on commercial sources. We can grow many of these herbs in our own gardens. Others we can seek out in the fields and roadsides, and gather prudently for our own use, being careful to leave enough of the plants so that they can propagate themselves. These wildlings are robust, but still we must treat them courteously. If we make friends among the country people where we vacation, as I recommended earlier, we can ask them to send us samples of the wild plants growing in their neighborhood. This is the sort of favor people love to do.

Herbs collected in this fashion have the advantages of being fresh and coming from a known source. For a plant is a fragile thing. Even dried, it will not keep forever. It deteriorates and loses much of its virtue. Dusty old herbs are almost worthless as medicines. I, myself, will only undertake to treat certain ailments during seasons when my stock of herbs is fresh and abundant. This is why I cannot be of help in emergencies or handle chronic diseases. But it is sometimes difficult to make a patient understand that this is not the season for celandine and that he will have to bide his time until the flower appears.

I have the same problems with my beauty preparations. There are times when my shop is out of certain creams. Some customers seem astonished when they are told that we are out of what they want because the stock of rose petals is used up. For I make it a policy to use only the products of my own gardens and fields. Then I know that my ingredients are the real thing, and are free of any chemicals.

You can follow the same policy. Gather your simples yourself, rather than buying sachets of unknown origin and dubious virtues. Look for plants on your country walks or on your weekend drives. Avoid picking plants from beside busy highways, where the vegetation is poisoned by car exhaust.

Observe the ways plants grow in the wild and you will have learned much about botanical sociology. For a field is a collectivity. If you want to grow some wild things in the rough bit of meadow behind your house, you must reproduce the conditions of the wilds, where variety and contrast reign. You will note that there are tall, strapping plants which send their stalks high and their roots deep, while there are other very small plants that hide beneath the tall ones, grateful for the moisture and shade, spreading their roots in the top layer of the soil. There are guardian plants that repel insects, and tender plants that require this protection. There are strongly scented plants and others with hardly any scent. There are plants that rejoice in sun and others that grow at the water's edge. The different characters and requirements of these plants complement and strengthen one another, just as vegetables do in a kitchen garden. The essential thing is to reproduce a favorable atmosphere for your various plants, a meadow in miniature.

Do not try to bring in foreign and exotic plants. They will not be happy in alien soil and you want only happy plants, for plants have to be happy to communicate their virtues. It is much the same with women. But if you observe these few conditions, your mixed planting can become a marvelous medical preserve.

Now let us go together on an herb-gathering expedition. For my father these expeditions were an ever-renewed joy and I grew up feeling it was a privilege to be allowed to go along. Sometimes one of Father's friends would join us. He was also a plant lover and bore the nickname of Caoulet, which in our Gascon dialect means "Little Cabbage." The implication was that he had the lore of plants in his blood. By trade, Caoulet was the bell-ringer in our village church. Morning, noon and evening he pulled on the bell ropes with all his might. The rest of the time he was at leisure and was always ready to go out to the fields with us.

I respected him, for he was obviously in the direct employ of the Lord. But the first time I ever went into his little house I was disappointed to find no other treasure inside than a pitcher of water on the table and a string of red onions and a few bunches of herbs hanging from the rafters. Caoulet lived sparely but reached an advanced age.

Nowadays I sometimes cover the same territory we used to comb, my father, Caoulet and I. For I have bought the woods of Lacassagne, which adjoins Gavarret, and the land serves as a source for most of my herbs. I have confidence in what grows here, out of the sound wild soil that has never been treated with chemicals. For me, the plants that grow in this bit of the world are the best.

I am very strict with the people I hire to pick for me. One of them, who wanted to impress me by his high production, ignored my orders and began going to certain places where the plant he was gathering was much more abundant than in my fields. But there was pollution there. When I learned what he had been doing, I dismissed him. I tell all my people, whether they are hired to pick at peak season or all through the year: "I am paying you for your time, not for the quantity you bring in. Do the best you can but do not go looking for plants outside my own grounds."

Serge, who supervises the other pickers, has been working for me for six years. His wife also pitches in at peak season. He knows that my rules are meant in earnest, and he tries to explain the reasons for them to the other pickers. At the height of summer I sometimes have a team of twenty to thirty people gathering for me, and scrupulosity becomes very important.

But sometimes I worry. Responsible workers are hard to find. Nor can the sound fields of Gavarret supply enough for my present needs, even if we pick from twenty-five to thirty sacks per day throughout the summer. Shall I send to the Pyrenees for celandine? For celandine carpets whole slopes there. But I prefer to find what I need at home. I dream of turning the whole region between Gavarret and Fleurance into a vast preserve of wild plants, where the nettles as well as the field flowers would all find their place.

But when I mention any such idea to the farmers, they look at me askance. Turn over their cultivated fields to the nettles? What decadence! But I have not given up on this dream. As with my campaign for organically-grown food, I hope to put across my point by the same gradual approach. I ask one man to lease me an acre of pasture land, another to give me rights to a patch of nettles. From another farmer I ask permission to use a hillside overgrown with ivy and heather. We draw up a contract. They will not lose.

For I do not want to import my herbs from Hungary and Czechoslovakia, as most herbalists do. I want a fresh supply daily for certain preparations, and I like to supervise the drying of others in the good open air under the good sun of my home village.

With herbs, there are no short cuts. They can take revenge for any indifference with which they are treated. Some herb teas we buy are quite dead from being shut up too long in their airtight packets. Others may be harmful because the herbs were gathered heaven knows where, from along busy highways or fields treated with chemicals. Therefore, before I present my recipes, I want to stipulate that the results are dependent on you yourself gathering the herbs mentioned. Nor is this requirement so unreasonable. It used to be a saying that the future belongs to him who wakes early. My feeling is that rising at dawn and going out into the fields to look for herbs, or into your own garden to pluck plants with the dew still on them, will do a great deal for your future, if not in terms of fortune, at least in terms of health. Which counts for more.

Herb-gathering is a meticulous art. The first thing we have to learn is to gather the flower, the leaf or the root at that moment in the day and the season when its valuable essences are at their best. This is what is known in herbalist terminology as "the balsamic moment."

The best hours are generally in the morning and the late afternoon. The foliage should be dry but the plant should not be sunscorched. Better do no gathering in rainy weather for your herbs are apt to mildew.

Flowers are fragile and fleeting. They should be picked almost as soon as they open in the springtime, before they have been pollinated. With some flowers only the petals are taken (rose, poppy, violet), while with others you take the entire flower when it is tiny (elderblossom, veronica). Certain plants have a very brief blossom time. Peach blossoms, for instance, last only a few days. Others go on flowering over a long interval—camomile, for instance—and you need not hurry to pick them.

Leaves are generally picked before the flowers appear, for afterwards the energy of the plant goes into the flowers. The exception to this rule is the aromatic herbs, for their active essences do not diminish during their flowering. Some aromatic plants can be gathered all through the year (parsley, thyme, rosemary, bay).

The larger leaves are plucked from the stalk (mallow, borage, bay), while with smaller leaves generally the whole stem is taken. We cut the stem some inches above ground, leaving the woody base behind to sprout again. For certain plants it is the stalks we want, and these are particularly rich in autumn when the rest of the plant has become inactive. An example of this is angelica.

Spring and fall are the proper times for gathering roots, for they are plump and juicy then. A sharp tug of the plant will in most cases uproot it. Then the root is carefully cut away and deposited in the gathering basket.

As I go along, I sort out the contents of my basket, discarding any spoiled plants, faded flowers or withered roots since only healthy material should be kept for medicinal use. Once I am home I arrange my pickings on screens so they will dry out evenly, and I often stir the plants so that every part of them will be exposed to the air.

Some of my screens are out in an open shed, others inside my herb house. The herb house is where I keep my stores of herbs; they are sheltered from the weather but are insured an ample supply of fresh air. The smell of the drying plants is particularly delightful, and I always feel a special joy in seeing the screens racked up one above the other and spread with a vast variety of plants, of varying shapes and shades of green.

If you have no shed, you can dry your herbs in your attic. The chief requirement is that the place be dry and airy. Sometimes the top of a cupboard will do. Spread it with clean paper and remember to turn your herbs occasionally. Never put your herbs into the oven to dry them quickly. That is a barbarous practice, for heat completely destroys the active properties of the herbs.

Learn to handle your herbs with tenderness, avoiding any motion that might bruise or break them. Pluck the leaves off by hand. Knives or any contact with metal is detrimental to them. Stir them often, so they may breathe. Clean them carefully: wash the earth off the roots and pat them dry. Do not use a chopping blade but rub the dried leaves between your fingers to powder them. They will repay you for this sort of kind treatment.

To know plants and understand their qualities you must become friends with them. Their friendship is not easy to win, but once won, it is long-lasting. Just as you must go to some pains to penetrate the psychology of children, so you must make an effort to grasp the nature of the various plants. Little by little you will discern their underlying laws.

In bygone times people would be guided by what was called the "signature" of plants. They would deduce the plants' properties from their form, their taste, their color. All plants with yellow juice, like rhubarb, were bitter but were useful for the liver, they concluded. Deep red was a sign of astringence: red roses, therefore, were so classified. White signified only weak medicinal action, while black or deep brown meant danger and poison (belladonna).

Nowadays we classify simples and vegetables by their family. Plants of the same group usually possess the same medicinal qualities. The cucurbitaceous plants (cucumbers, squashes, melons) are laxative. The cruciferous plants (carrots, wild carrots) are stimulants and antiscorbutants. The rosaceous plants (roses, hawthorn) are astringent and tonic. The labiate plants (mint, marjoram, thyme) are stimulant and sudoriferous. And so on. This does not mean that any plant that bears a close resemblance to one we know is necessarily a close relative and has the same properties. Nature is full of false doubles. Beware of the hemlock, which looks remarkably like parsley!

This little guide to simples cannot begin to cover the great number of useful plants growing all about us. It is not necessary to become an expert on the entire subject. If you know only a single plant, gather it and put it to use. As you become acquainted with the more common herbs, learn what each can do and soon you will have formed that happy intimacy with plants which will yield you both pleasure and health.

In human friendship we come to know not only the strong points of our friends but their faults and weaknesses as well. It is the same with plants. I will not conceal the dangers of an imprudent use of certain capricious plants. An example is the celandine. This dainty yellow flower has strong properties out of proportion to its size. I use it in homeopathic doses in many of my preparations. Yet in a larger dose it can be harmful. Above all, it must never be taken internally.

My father used to pay close attention to the ways of animals with plants. They seemed to know which plants acted as purgatives and would seek out special herbs whenever they had trouble with their digestions. Even our cats, pampered house pets though they were, had enough wild instinct in them to take to the fields when they felt the need for some tonic. Work-weary horses and donkeys would crop the bitter leaves of dandelion, centaury, pimpernel. Conversely, young and vigorous beasts would shun these herbs. Milking cows and young animals at the start of the mating season would nibble eagerly on fenugreek, wild fennel and meadow saffron, all of which stimulate the sex glands.

Good pasture land contains a large assortment of herbs, and the animals choose what they require according to their physical state. The hedgerows furnish them with more variety. Country veterinarians will still recommend this plant or that to restore an ailing animal's balance.

The older country people manage to look after their beasts fairly well with the material at hand. During a difficult calving, they will give the cow an infusion of sage leaves and juniper. A cow with digestive troubles is given a good bunch of gorse, while a horse whose blood is thin is doctored with heather. Couch grass is the traditional remedy for kidney stones in horses, and a farmer will go a long distance to pick some if he has none in his own fields. It seems to me that mothers should also know such simple herbal remedies to administer to their children in case of fever or an upset stomach. Of course, neither farmer nor mother should delay calling a doctor when the case is serious.

Another lesson we might relearn is the importance of the symbolic gesture in relation to health. A child, I think, feels more gratitude toward his mother when she brings him a glass of steaming herbal tea than when she hands him a tablet out of a box. Similarly, the hard-working husband appreciates his wife's efforts to maintain his health with good food tastefully prepared and attractively served. This is far more reassuring than having to swallow a few vitamin pills every day. Our hearts respond better to simples and to those who offer them to us than to pills and capsules. And this intuitive response is the very thing which in many cases helps the body rally and throw off its illness. Thus, if these herbal remedies do no more than bring pleasure to the eyes, the nostrils, the lips and the heart, they would have accomplished a great deal.

But their power does not end with their sense appeal. That is only how they win our trust. They must prove their claims. So since we do not have any professors of herbalism, the herbs themselves must speak their pieces. Let us call them up, one by one, and let each tell us what it can do.

Parsley and Chervil

Roman gladiators would eat parsley before going into combat. Their strength and courage was supposed to show an immediate rise.

In our day parsley is popular enough. When your greengrocer wants to be especially amiable, he will present you with a little bunch of parsley. It is the best gift he could offer, a veritable bouquet of health. Yet too often parsley is treated as a mere ornament, as when we see it trimming a calf's head in a butcher shop window. In restaurants, too, the main dish is often decorated with clusters of parsley, with the result that the garnish is pushed aside uneaten. It is a great mistake to use parsley this way. It should be chopped fine and sprinkled over the food so that it will be eaten without fail.

Parsley is one of the easiest herbs to raise and belongs in every garden. Use it liberally—your cooking and your health will be noticeably improved. Why not also put in some chervil, parsley's mate in both appearance and virtues? Some people prefer planting chervil because there is less danger of confounding it with the dangerous hemlock plant that sometimes crops up in gardens as a weed. But there is an easy way to tell the good herb from the bad, despite the deceptive resemblance. If you rub a bit of hemlock leaf, it gives off an unpleasant smell like that of cat's urine.

Both parsley and chervil enhance salads, omelettes and soups. They dry well and are useful in the winter. Remember that of all plants, these are among the richest in vitamin C. Parsley also has stimulating properties. It is recommended for jaundice and for all liver ailments, for cellulite, gout and rheumatism.

Besides its well-known uses in cooking, parsley is good steeped in warm milk or made into a tea. My grandmother Sophie was a firm believer in parsley and could hardly have cooked without it. I remember her Pantagruelian fare on the occasion of some village festival. Of course, we started off with a goose liver *pâté*, the famous *foie gras* of Gascony. The main dish was roast chicken and pigeon, with plenty of parsley in the stuffing. Accompanying this were mushrooms sautéed with garlic and dusted with parsley and mountains of tasty crêpes (Grandmother always put parsley into the batter). We finished up with delicate custards and a succession of other desserts including Gascon-style apple tart. Yet after this repast no one ever complained of indigestion. It is significant that after dinner Grandmother brewed a monster pot of parsley tea and pressed a cup on everyone. "For your stomach," she would say. No one refused.

If you do not feel attracted by the thought of parsley tea, I would suggest that you add a good bunch of parsley to your homemade vegetable juice. You can blend an ambrosial drink from ripe tomatoes, carrots and celery, spiked with a dash of lemon juice and a handful of parsley.

In bygone days wet nurses used to salve their breasts with a paste made of parsley to keep the milk from gushing out. Parsley also makes a soothing unguent against insect bites. Rub it vigorously over the swelling.

I myself like to use parsley against conjunctivitis and other eye inflammations. Steep the chopped leaves in boiling water, cool to body temperature, and apply the solution with an eye cup. It soothes the burning sensation and acts as disinfectant.

A similar solution applied to the face with a cotton wad morning and night diminishes ruddiness and cleans the complexion.

Thyme

The good King Charlemagne, ever mindful of the welfare of his people, set down all sorts of instructions for the conduct of the country in a series of decrees known as the Capitularies. He did not think it beneath his royal dignity to command that aromatic herbs be planted in the gardens of monasteries and his royal estates. For herbs glorified whatever dish they were added to, and the king wanted his people to eat well.

Governments today do not pass laws concerning the growing of herbs. I find this a great pity. All I can do is make my recommendations, and hope that my readers will do the rest. One recommendation is that every garden, large or small, contain a clump of thyme, for it is a precious herb with almost more uses than I can enumerate.

Even in antiquity it was known that certain aromatic herbs had strong antiseptic powers and could quell infection. Thyme was one such herb. In olden days, when people had no other protection against epidemics and plagues, they tried using the aromatic herbs in every possible way, rubbing their bodies with the leaves and burning the plants to banish miasmas.

Nowadays we know they were on the right track. Thyme contains an antiseptic known as thymol, which is even more powerful than phenol, long considered the best of the antibacterial agents. Thymol is a camphorous substance extracted from thyme, and it serves as base for a great number of pharmaceutical products— syrups, pomades, balms and lotions. Thymol is even used to wash a wound after an amputation.

To be sure, in our time plague no longer stalks the land and even amputations have become a rarity. Medicine has made great advances and we no longer need to depend on thyme for such drastic uses. Yet is this any reason for forgoing its benefactions? During an epidemic of flu, for instance, we notice that some people succumb to the virus, while others in the same family or same surroundings seem able to withstand it. In hospitals, doctors and nurses who work in an atmosphere rife with germs are usually immune to them. How can that be? It is a question of predisposition, we are told. Some people are prone to a disease, others have natural resistance to it. But in fact, such resistance is acquired. The secret is to maintain general good health and to create a climate within the body that repels harmful microorganisms. Diet plays a great part in this, and the seasonings we use are especially pertinent. Thus garlic is a prime germicide, as are the aromatic herbs. A person whose body is impregnated with these scents can sometimes pass through veritable pestholes without coming to harm.

I do not mean to suggest that you fall back on your bouquet of thyme when your next-door neighbor or co-worker comes down with the flu. Emergency measures of that sort are no great help, I'm afraid. What I want to say is this: If you use thyme in all its forms, making it part of your life, you will be spared many a bout of flu and other miseries (though not all) and you will preserve your health. Perhaps you will not even be aware of what you owe your good fortune to, for it is difficult to take account of what one has been spared.

Make a habit, then, of using thyme—either garden thyme or the smaller, finer wild thyme so beloved of rabbits which you can bring back from a country excursion. First of all, never forget to include a branch of thyme in the bouquet of herbs you drop into your soups or stews. Include thyme in your stuffings and salad dressings, and sprinkle it liberally over any grilled meats. Thyme is much used in warm climates because food there is more exposed to spoilage. Have you ever wondered how marinated meats used to stay fresh in the days before refrigeration? The marinating mixture always contained a goodly quantity of thyme and this was enough to discourage the microbes.

Make a thyme tea by simmering a branch of the herb in a pint of water. This refreshing beverage can be drunk three or four times a day, between meals and at breakfast. Sweetened with honey, it is particularly delicious. In Provence they use wild thyme this way and call it shepherd's tea.

I employ the same brew to treat stubborn intestinal infections, flus, colds and tonsillitis. I cannot presume to say how many of my patients have avoided these nasty illnesses by their faithful use of thyme, but I am always singing its praises.

Used externally, thyme is a dependable disinfectant. It will even draw out the poison of snake venom. Cuts and gashes will never fester if washed with an infusion of thyme. A big bunch of thyme in the daily bath will alleviate many skin diseases. Oil of thyme, sold under a number of trade names, used in the bath will bring relief to rheumatism and arthritis. Since such baths are highly stimulating, they are also recommended for low-energy children, lymphatics and convalescents.

Chopped thyme will make a comforting poultice for rheumatism. Warm the mash and apply it to the painful area.

An inhalation of menthol or eucalyptus bought at the drug-store will be much improved by an added pinch of thyme.

Lastly, if you have a tendency to develop mouth or throat sores, this disinfectant mouthwash will be of help: Chop 100 grams of thyme and steep for several days in a pint of pure alcohol. Use daily, applying the mixture with toothbrush to the teeth and gums.

Rosemary

This little shrub, which grows wild throughout southern Europe, had its moment of glory when it bestowed youth and beauty upon a queen. Legend has it that Queen Elizabeth of Hungary, already seventy-two and crippled with gout and rheumatism, was given a secret lotion which so restored her charms that the King of Poland fell head over heels in love with her and insisted on mak-ing her his wife. All this took place in the fourteenth century, and the miraculous lotion was supposedly given to the queen by an angel. Of course, queens would rather receive angelic gifts than old wives' recipes, and if the queen was as infirm as the legend makes her, the effects of the lotion were indeed miracu-lous. Nevertheless, the "toilet water of the Queen of Hungary," as the lotion has since been called, contained some sprigs of rose-mary steeped in pure alcohol, along with other herbs like mar-joram and lavender whose antirheumatoid properties are well known today. It is not so astonishing, then, that the queen de-rived a great deal of benefit from it.

The toilet water of the Queen of Hungary was passed along through the ages, along with the legend and the attribution to the angel. The Duchess of Sévigné swore by it: "I am mad about it," she wrote to her daughter. "It is a balm for all my griefs."

Nor was she alone in her enthusiasm. Since her day, "Hungarian water" has been employed not only to alleviate gout and rheuma-tism but also against fainting spells and languor. Older ladies have looked to it to revive their attractions and gentlemen no longer in their prime have looked to it to revive their failing powers.

Rosemary therefore, has a reputation for miracles, nor is this totally unjustified, for the herb has a wide spectrum of powers. It is effective against rheumatism, paralysis, weakness of the limbs and attacks of vertigo. It alleviates nervous conditions and respiratory troubles, corrects malfunction of the liver and gall bladder, and even helps with potency disturbances.

All this is reason enough to give rosemary a place of honor in your cooking. Include it in your sauces and your gravies, and sprinkle it generously over pork roasts and leg of lamb. Certain honeys of the Midi are made largely from the blossom of rosemary, and partake not only of the fragrance of the herb but also of its many virtues.

Like thyme, rosemary makes a healthful tea that can be drunk throughout the day with tangible benefit. For those who like a heartier beverage, I recommend rosemary wine. Steep 50 grams of rosemary in your favorite Bordeaux for a few days, and enjoy a glass of this with every meal. It has a strong tonic effect.

For external use, you may not wish to go through all the complicated procedures followed by the Queen of Hungary (according to the prescripts of her angel), but try a sprig of rosemary in your bath water. You had better do this in the morning, for such a bath is highly stimulating (some even find it aphrodisiac) and is not conducive to peaceful sleep. I recommend it especially for sickly children and older people with flagging energy.

A handful of rosemary boiled for fifteen minutes in a quart of water makes a good poultice to apply against the pain of rheumatism.

Extract of rosemary is a favorite ingredient in many pharmaceutical and cosmetic products.

Sage

Why should a man die, who has sage growing in his garden? This proverb, according the highest homage to sage, was coined in the Middle Ages in Salerno, one of the most celebrated medical centers of the time. Actually, the plant's virtues had been recognized far earlier by the Romans, who referred to it as the "the sacred herb" or "*salvia salviatrix*" (the herb that saves).

Thus it is scarcely surprising that sage should have been an ingredient in so many panaceas of the past. But its most drama-tic use was in the so-called Vinegar of the Four Robbers. When Toulouse was struck by the terrible plague of 1630, four robbers went about the city, entering infected houses and taking what they pleased from the dead and dying. Despite the enormous risk, they were able to resist contagion. Finally the authorities managed to seize them. Condemned to death, the men were offered clemency if they would disclose their secret remedy against the plague. The four were willing to buy their lives on this basis. Their deposition may still be found in the archives of Toulouse. They had compounded a vinegar steeped with sage, thyme, lavender, rosemary and several other aromatic herbs which, as we now know, are strong germicides, and rubbed this mixture over their entire bodies.

A century later an epidemic of plague hit Marseilles and an-other band saw their chance for theft and looting. They protected themselves with the vinegar of their predecessors, improving on it somewhat by adding a few more herbs. The herbalists of Mar-seilles also remembered this old formula, to which they added garlic, a beloved item in those parts and known since Galen's day as an excellent antiseptic. In this form the Vinegar of the Four Robbers remained in the pharmaceutical register until the end of the nineteenth century, and we may presume that it proved its efficacy many, many times. It was even offered commercially —a M. Malle, a licensed vinegar-maker, manufactured it accord-ing to the ancient formula.

Like its fellow labiates thyme and rosemary, sage possesses strong antiseptic properties. Its other properties are equally im-portant. It reduces night sweating, for which reason sage is recom-mended for people recovering from a high fever. It will arrest an incipient case of flu. Since sage has a regulating effect on the hormones, it is useful for girls in their puberty, for pregnant women and for women with menopause problems. Sage soothes a troublesome cough and tempers stomach pains. Above all, it is a tonic and stimulating, which is why it should be a preferred food for neurasthenics. On the same score, it should be avoided by those whose temperments are already too highly charged.

Sage is invaluable in the kitchen, adding its unique flavor to sauces and stuffings as well as to grilled meats. It is especially compatible with mild-flavored meats like pork, and makes them more digestible. In Provence a sprig of sage is always added to the soup, along with the equally indispensable fried garlic. Keep this in mind when you attempt one of the country soups that are currently coming back into fashion. Also remember that although sage grows wild on the stony uplands of Provence and the Lozere district, it is perfectly happy growing in the kitchen garden.

Therefore establish a few of these pretty gray-green plants where you will have them conveniently at hand for cooking purposes. Gather the fresh sprigs, what herbalists call the flowering tips, where the plant's active essences are most concentrated, for use in fragrant teas.

You can concoct a healthful after-dinner drink by steeping 100 grams of sage for a week in a quart of wine. A tiny glass of this taken at the end of a meal will do wonders for the digestion. It is also an excellent tonic for the convalescent.

For mulled wine, try a pinch of dried sage in place of the usual cinnamon.

Sage has a good number of external uses. Prepare a decoction of sage by boiling a handful of the leaves in a quart of water for ten minutes. Strain and use either for washing wounds, as a gargle or a vaginal douche. In all cases, it is a dependable antiseptic.

A bouquet of sage thrown into your bath water will, like rosemary, give your ablutions a tonic and even aphrodisiac quality. Such baths are excellent in the morning for people of low energy. However, highly charged people had better avoid them.

Savory

My father always had special respect for savory. He used to tell me: "You see, my boy, it is one of those herbs that brings us happiness."

One day I overheard a conversation between my father and the village priest in which the abbé mentioned that in olden days monks were forbidden to plant savory and rocket in their gardens. Hidden behind the door, I puzzled over this enigmatic piece of information.

Later on, I understood that these so-called herbs of happiness were those plants that were favorable to love.

Folk etymology traces the French word for savory, *sarriete*, to satyr. This may be sheer invention. Nevertheless, if the Greeks attached some meaning of this sort to the fragrant herb, they must have had good reason. Just like the licentious satyrs who played their pipes and disported endlessly with the nymphs of antiquity, men who nibbled on savory found that their amorous abilities increased tenfold. The same effect is observable in donkeys, for they, too, know the herb and are very partial to it. In fact, in my part of the country, savory is also called "donkey's pepper."

Hence I include savory in my love philters, along with celandine, fenugreek and cow parsnip. When I read accounts of what used to go into the lover philters of bygone days, I have to smile; my mixtures are so simple by comparison.

I have never played with powdered spanish fly, which the Borgias used to blend into their concoctions and with which Mme. de Montespan plied Louis XV to arouse his ardor. There is also the story of the Marquis de Sade's offering a group of guests chocolates containing spanish fly, in order to test the merits of the substance (which is actually the ground-up bodies of a type of beetle). A full-scale orgy ensued, so our indefatigible experimenter must have been convinced the product had all the effects claimed for it.

But I am a simple fellow, a man of the soil. I merely counsel the wife who worries over her husband's indifference to fill her pepper mill with savory, and grind it generously over her husband's steak—and hers, too, if she is so minded. This way, she will be sure that the herb is eaten, not pushed aside as so often happens with garnishing.

I cannot promise you that a pinch of savory eaten once in your lifetime will bring you to the brink of an orgy. I simply say that a couple who over the years enjoy a stimulating diet comprising a goodly amount of garlic, onion, celery, fennel, sage and savory have a pretty good chance of experiencing conjugal happiness.

Since savory also aids digestion, it is wise to throw a sprig into your stews. It goes especially well with game. Dried beans and peas, which are somewhat hard to digest, will benefit from the addition of savory.

My father, who was a firm believer in the principle of osmosis, (as I am), made an invigorating lotion by boiling a handful of savory and a handful of fenugreek in a quart of water. With this he would rub the spinal columns of patients who complained of enervation. After a number of such treatments, the patients would turn up, looking very jaunty, to thank my father for restoring their virility.

Now, some forty years later, I still rely on the same ingredients for one of my revitalizing creams meant for massaging the spinal column.

You can treat savory much as you do thyme, sage and rosemary, for all these plants are of the same family, and throw a handful of it into your bath. Whether absorbed by way of the mouth or by way of the skin, savory always has the same effect.

Bay Leaf

From time immemorial laurel wreaths have crowned the brows of poets, generals, and emperors. Why was laurel chosen for this honor? Because the noble laurel tree was sacred to Apollo, god of the sun and of the arts.

Nowadays laurel has been somewhat downgraded. It appears more often in soup as bay leaf (the dried leaf of the laurel) than on the brow of heroes. Bay leaves are essential to the classic *bouquet garni*, and are also used for curing country hams in France. An enormous bunch of the leaves is hung in the chimney and the ham suspended above. As the smoke passes through the bay leaves, it carries their fragrance into the ham. Moreover, the antiseptic qualities of bay help preserve the meat. For this same reason, bay leaves are part of every pickling solution. In bygone days people would burn branches of bay during epidemics to protect their houses against the surrounding miasmas. Bay leaves, then, have many of the same qualities as thyme, sage and rosemary. But the laurel tree has the advantage of size. You would have to pick a great sack of thyme to obtain the equivalent of a single branch of bay.

Besides the distinctive flavor the bay leaf imparts to food, it also stimulates digestive action. Hence it is a highly valuable condiment on many accounts.

But I must warn you against resting on your laurels. For while the common laurel has all these praiseworthy properties, some members of the laurel family are dangerous: the oleander, the cherry laurel and several other types.

In the past cooks might have given a faint almond taste to custards by dropping a single leaf of the cherry laurel into the milk. But our grandmothers were prudent and knew what they were about. It was always one leaf, not two, for two would have been enough to poison the whole family.

In fact, cherry laurel is effective in homeopathic doses against coughs, palpitations, vomiting and stomach cramps. But it contains prussic acid, which in only slightly larger doses is a poison. Similarly, oleander leaves are also poisonous, yet from them we extract an excellent heart stimulant.

Prudence has always been a key principle of the science of plants.

Basil

Basil has acquired a number of different names—ranging all the way from "royal herb" to "cobbler's orange." Though it originally came from India, the plant is by now totally acclimated to the Mediterranean lands. In Provence we consider it a household necessity, and dry great bunches of basil by hanging them head down from the ceiling beams. We make a soup of basil, which is known as *soupe au pistou,* and whose fame has spread far beyond our region.

In the past basil was prescribed for epilepsy and madness. Of course, nowadays if your child should prove epileptic I would urge you to put him under care of a good neurologist. But if your child should be of a nervous disposition, have trouble sleeping and show a tendency to dizziness and headaches, I would suggest that you put a good *soupe au pistou* on the dinner table several times a week. Its calming effects will soon be apparent. As for your husband, he will be happy to be served duck with basil, which is one of the glories of gastronomy. Moreover, the addition of the basil leaves makes the fowl highly digestible, for basil fends off stomach spasms and intestinal infections.

You may make a fragrant tea with basil, as with the other aromatic herbs. Drunk in the evening, it promotes sound sleep and a good digestion. But you should keep in mind which of the herbal teas are calming and which are stimulating. Just as you would not brew a pot of linden tea for breakfast and coffee in the late evening, so you must not confuse your herbs and drink them at inappropriate times of the day. Sage is good in the morning and calming basil in the evening. If you reverse this order, you may find your whole day turned topsy-turvy.

Tarragon

My grandmother Sophie put it into everything. Whenever I had hiccups, she would run to the garden, come back with a sprig of tarragon and say: "Here, my little one, chew this up, the naughty hiccups will go away."

And the hiccups would indeed subside. I have since discovered that tarragon regulates stomach gas, controls flatulence, acidity and various stomach and intestinal disorders.

In addition, "the little dragon," as the plant used to be called, has a spicy flavor that greatly enhances every kind of food. Tarragon can easily take the place of salt, pepper and vinegar, if you should be without these at the moment or if your doctor has proscribed them. When patients complain to me of the insipidity of their salt-free diets, I tell them: "It needn't be a problem. Sprinkle some tarragon on your salad and beefsteak. Try tarragon chicken, one of the easiest dishes to prepare. You will not only be eating splendidly, but along with pleasing your palate you will be helping your stomach and delicate intestines to mend."

As for those who are not on any diet, I would equally urge them to sprinkle tarragon on their salads and *crudités*. A vinegar is also greatly improved by steeping some tarragon in it. There are a few good brands of this on the market, and very attractive the bottles are, with the sprig of tarragon floating in the midst of the rose-colored vinegar.

When country people put up pickled gherkins, or some of the other favorite sweet-and-sours (cherries, green beans, tiny onions, pickled cauliflower, carrot sticks and the delicious Gascon-style blue plums) they always include a sprig of tarragon in the jar. This neutralizes the effect of the vinegar upon the stomach.

If you have eaten too heavily and foresee bad consequences, have a glass of tarragon tea. Then you will not suffer from a rumbling stomach the day after a gala dinner.

Marjoram

> *The king's son fell in love with me*
> *With my* sabots *on,*
> *And made me a present of a bunch*
> *Of marjoram,*
> *With my* sabots *on.*

I used to sing this song when I was little. And since I, too, clattered around in *sabots*, I used to puzzle over the song's meaning, in the manner of small children who sense significance behind simple words but lack the essential clue to the riddle. Why, I asked my father, did the king's son make a present of marjoram? Was it a royal gift, because of the loveliness of the flower or the velvet quality of the leaves? Or was there something else about the plant?

My father replied that it was because marjoram calms all griefs, even the pangs of love.

The oregano used so much in Italian cooking, included in all their sauces and sprinkled lavishly on pizzas, is simply another form of marjoram. To be sure, it is stronger and more pungent, but then passions are stronger in Italy than in France.

I have spent much of my life making discoveries, noticing parallels and testing premises. But since I am not a sophisticated man, I always try to arrive at the simplest formulation of my findings, with the result that I am often not taken seriously.

Thus when a man comes to me, deeply convinced of the magnitude of his problem, and tells me: "Monsieur Mességué, I am devoured by passion. I cannot sleep at night. What should I do?" I am apt to answer: "Eat pizzas." And I say so in good faith. But the man goes away thinking me a charlatan. Yet my answer was perfectly serious, if a bit elliptic. My mind simply leaped to that pinch of marjoram, or oregano, with which pizzas are always powdered, and which would assure my client a good night's sleep. Then again, I was thinking that a good way to assuage an unhappy passion is to substitute a little ordinary *joie de vivre* for it—and such *joie de vivre* is often abundantly present in small Italian restaurants. Hence I would also advise those who suffer from various nervous tics and digestive spasms to eat pizza. So you see, I am still clattering around "with my *sabots* on" like the peasant girl in the song.

I might also answer: "Have a glass of marjoram tea in the evening before bedtime." Would people accept this advice more readily? The underlying principle is the same. Marjoram is an excellent tranquilizer and as such I recommend it in every form, in cooking, in an infusion, as a gargle, as a vapor, in the bath and in poultices. People with rheumatism should apply marjoram compresses to the painful areas. People with colds should set a handful of marjoram boiling in an open saucepan and inhale the vapors. They may then profitably drink the same brew. Singers with sensitive throats should drink marjoram tea sweetened with honey. But a word of warning: in too strong a dose marjoram can become a stupefying drug.

Mint

The markets in Arab lands smell delightfully of mint, for there are always a number of little donkeys about with bunches of mint in their panniers. The scent of the mint dispels the flies and mosquitoes, which would otherwise be swarming over the food. In very hot weather one will see people walking about with bunches of fresh mint in their hands at which they sniff constantly, as though the scent alone kept down the temperature.

The perfume of mint tea wafts from mosaic-covered palaces as well as from the simplest of houses. Serving mint tea is nearly a sacred rite, as well as a wise precaution. For these lands are still subject to epidemics and the prevailing heat favors the spread of microbes. Having mint constantly about is a health measure, for mint is a strong antiseptic. It was one of the ingredients of the Vinegar of the Four Robbers, which I have already described. So mint is prized in these hot countries not only for its perfume and bracing, cooling quality, but also because folk wisdom recognizes its medicinal powers.

Mint is used all over the world in a vast number of ways. In Asia it is added to pilafs and pastries, while in the United States it is indispensable in certain cocktails and tall drinks. The English can scarecly eat their mutton without an accompanying mint sauce, while the French and Swiss are partial to mint teas. If you have fresh mint available, I would advise you to try some in your salads. It adds an exquisite note.

The commercial dried mint for use in teas is a cultivated type of peppermint. There are many other varieties, both wild and cultivated, with subtle differences in flavor. All possess the same properties to a greater or lesser degree. Gather great bunches of wild mint just before it comes into flower, dry it and use it freely. Simply having the bouquets hanging in your kitchen is a delight to the senses. Insects will be noticeably absent from the room in which mint is drying.

The mint tea you drink merely for pleasure has more virtues than I can list. I will mention only the more important ones. First is its antiseptic properties. Then there are its benefits to the digestion. Mint is a balm for the entire digestive tract, regulating stomach, liver, gall bladder and intestines. It is effective against stomach gas, stomach spasms, vomiting, liver complaints, intestinal parasites and colic.

People with a tendency to travel sickness should always equip themselves with peppermint drops.

A drop of essence of mint on a sugar cube is a standard remedy against dizziness, for the mint stimulates the heart and the nervous system. This tonic property makes mint tea an excellent drink for intellectuals. It also counters the enervation of hot climates.

I therefore would advise you to have your mint tea in the morning or in the course of the day, but not at bedtime, when it can induce a bit of insomnia. If you want to avail yourself of its digestive properties after too rich a dinner, mix it with linden, which is a calming herb. Your steaming glass of linden-mint tea will do you good, for the linden neutralizes the excitation induced by the mint. The alchemy of herbal teas is a fine art, but not too difficult to learn. You might also top off a hearty dinner with a mint-flavored dessert, which again would aid digestion.

There are innumerable commercial products based on mint: syrups, liqueurs, candies, lozenges, toothpastes, salves, etc. The antiseptic qualities of mint render it useful in all sorts of respiratory medicines. Menthol, so effective for opening blocked respiratory passages, is an extract of the mint plant. Should you come down with a cold and have no menthol product in your medicine chest, take a good pinch of your home-dried mint and cook up an infusion. While it is boiling, hold a towel, tent-like, over your head to capture all the vapors and breathe in the steam.

Applied externally, mint has a certain anesthetic effect. Children sometimes make a game of breathing hard while sucking on peppermint drops. The result is a sensation of intense cold which for a few moments resembles the numbness caused by a local anesthetic. More serious advantage may be taken of this analgesic property of mint. You can soothe a toothache by a drop of essence of mint on the sensitive spot. For a headache, dip a towel into an infusion of mint (a handful of mint leaves boiled ten minutes in a quart of water) and lay this warm compress on your brow. Similar compresses will lessen the pain of rheumatism until you can apply some mentholated rub to the affected areas. New mothers can reduce the swelling of their breasts with applications of fresh mint leaves, softened by being dipped into boiling water.

To come to the last of its virtues, mint has the reputation of being a potent aphrodisiac. One thing is certain: mint regulates the sexual functions of both men and women and lends zest to the games of love. Is the heady perfume of the mint the significant factor? I do not know, but in any case mint has always been included, in larger or smaller doses, in formulas for love potions. During my travels in the lands of the Thousand and One Nights I have detected among the perfumes drifting from the palaces of emirs and pashas a strong admixture of mint and I have wondered if these princes of Araby were not all masters of the science of herbs.

Nettles

We have a phrase in French: "To throw into the nettles," which means to discard something we no longer care for. But for my part, I would throw into the nettles what I cared for most. Though people regard nettles as a weed, I consider them one of the most valuable of plants. I have constituted myself the protector of nettles and have given strict orders to my farmers not to disturb these purple-blossomed plants which tend to spring up at the foot of a wall or a hedgerow. I also send out pickers to gather great sacks of nettles in their favorite locations, on the edge of ponds and in boggy places where nothing else will grow.

Everyone can lay in an ample supply of nettles, for here is a plant we all recognize, if only because we were warned against it when we were children. To be sure, nettles sting, but that is no reason to avoid them—only you must wear gloves when you pick them. My father, who handled all plants with instinctive gentleness, knew how to gather nettles without gloves by reaching for them from below. I am grateful to him for teaching me how to behave toward plants so that even the prickliest of them became my friends.

So if you should forget to take along your botany book on your country outing or picnic, you can at least come back with some nettles.

In olden days men would prove their bravery by flinging themselves into a bed of nettles. Not only was this an act of stoicism that added greatly to the standing of the man in question, but there were personal benefits had from it—the sting of the nettles would stimulate the circulation. In the country, when children come home with their legs all red and swollen from an encounter with the prickly plant, they are usually told: "Be glad. Because of this, you won't have rheumatism later on."

To this day there are people who will throw themselves into the nettles and claim they enjoy the sensation. I can personally vouch for one such case, the cavalry officer in Gavarret, the inveterate skirt-chaser who lived to be a hundred. He used to roll in the nettles the way some people scrub themselves with loofahs. Classical texts contain many references to this rough form of massage. Petronius, for instance, describes a priestess who would restore men to vigor by beating them with a bunch of nettles "above the navel, about the loins and across the buttocks, for in old men this part of the body is cold as the snow."

Following the same principle, Rabelais advised rubbing the backside with sea holly. (The sea holly is another hairy-leafed plant closely related to thistle.) Moreover, it used to be thought that whipping the body with nettles was a way to make certain diseases like measles and scarlet fever break through the surface.

Ovid, in his *Art of Love*, offers the recipe for a cunning love philter to which is added, at the last moment, a pinch of nettle seed. Is this only a metaphor for adding something stinging to the admixture of elements that lead to love?

I myself have a somewhat more homely use for nettles. I use them to medicate my old dogs who suffer, as so many older animals do, from rheumatism. For I always let my animals live out their natural span. When animals have spent their entire lives at my side, I cannot make myself pronounce their death sentence simply because they have grown somewhat ailing with the years. I also rescue other dogs who have been turned out of their homes because of their age and infirmities.

Thus my country place has gradually become a refuge for old dogs, and I make up medications for them much as I do for my human patients. So I will go out on a fine morning and pick a good mess of nettles from a nearby ditch. On the way back I will gather a bunch of celandine and step into the kitchen garden to choose a well-grown cabbage. I then chop up my harvest and set it to soak in rain water for two or three days. For I always have a supply of rain water on hand, gathering it in a wooden tub set under the eaves of the house, just as my father used to do. I then take this liquid and rub my old dogs with it, especially in the places that ache. As a result of this treatment, they last a few more years.

If you should find nettles springing up at the edge of your garden, do not destroy them with herbicides. Rather, water them and leave them in peace. According to Professor Pfeiffer, who has made a long study of the affinities among various plants, a row of nettles growing near aromatic and medicinal herbs substantially increases their content of beneficial oils.

Moreover, your nettle patch will provide you with some delicious dishes: nettle soup and creamed nettles, both of which rank among the most delicate and healthful foods you can serve. Treat the nettles just as you would spinach or other greens (in fact, they surpass spinach in their mineral content). After a moment's cooking they lose their prickliness and will be soft as velvet to the tongue. Nettles are an excellent depurative and diuretic.

Nettle tea is good for rheumatism. I give bowls of it to my dogs and they lap it as though they knew its virtues, animals having infallible instincts in this matter. In this form, nettles have a direct effect on the circulatory system and can arrest hemorrhages, quiet violent menstruation and nosebleeds, and heal bleeding hemorrhoids. The same infusion can be used as a gargle for sore throat and a wash for such skin conditions as eczema, acne and herpes. I use nettles in some of my beauty creams. Would my lady clients be startled to know that they owe their glowing complexions to stinging nettles?

Celandine

Since we have stepped out of the confines of the kitchen garden, let us go into the fields and make the acquaintance of that invaluable herb celandine.

"It is the best herb of all," my father used to say, "Or the most cruel."

According to legend, celandine makes the man who is going to die weep, while he who is going to be cured begins to sing.

The plant has many folk names—nightingale herb, goatweed, wart flower.

It is nothing special to look at—a small modest plant with a bright yellow flower. Break the stem and an orange juice trickles out. This juice is extremely bitter-tasting, which should serve as a warning not to eat it. Let me emphasize this warning. Whatever rare virtues celandine may possess, it is only for external use.

One day a letter came to me from a patient reporting that he had made infusions of the various herbs I had sent him and was feeling ever so much better. I had meant my package of herbs to be used for hand and foot baths and had included explicit directions to that effect. The patient had simply not read these instructions. I was appalled. My herb mixture had contained celandine, which in a large dose is a deadly poison. I could only conclude that my patient might ail in a number of ways but had a strong stomach.

I have planted a row of celandine on my grounds, placing it against the wall of a stone outbuilding because celandine seems to like the presence of stone. I notice that neither my horse, nor my donkey nor my geese ever take a nip of the plant. They deliberately avoid that side of the shed. As usual, animals are instinctively aware of this sort of danger.

In common with many other poisonous plants, celandine attracted interest in ancient times and there are many legends surrounding the plant. Because of the yellow color of its flower the alchemists included celandine in many of their formulas for making gold. Even its Latin name is a reference to supernatural qualities: *coeli donum* (gift of heaven).

Celandine was reputed to repel the plague and to restore sight to the blind. Its name "nightingale herb" came from the belief that the mother nightingale always placed a drop of the sap in the eyes of nestlings to sharpen their sight. As a matter of fact, there is a basis for this story, for the sap, diluted with water, is used as an eyewash against conjunctivitis.

Three or four applications of the orange sap upon a wart will make the wart disappear—hence its name wart flower. It is equally effective against corns and callouses.

According to the theory of signatures (which in previous ages played a large part in medical thinking), the yellow color of the flower meant that celandine was an agent against jaundice and all diseases of the liver and bile. There is no support for the general theory today—we know how faulty such associative reasoning can be—but in the case of celandine the supposition happens to be correct. Celandine is indeed useful against jaundice and other liver troubles. In homeopathic doses, which should be carefully supervised, celandine tea is a valuable purgative and diuretic and a remedy for bladder stones. In addition, it has soporific qualities that calm stomach spasms. Hence there are those who prescribe celandine for these purposes. However, I myself am cautious in this respect and prefer to restrict celandine to external uses only.

Pimpernel

The ancients made heavy use of pimpernel, for they considered it to have a direct influence on the blood. Hence, its other name of *sanguisorbe*.

It grows wild in our fields, preferring rich, moist soil. Pick great baskets of it, as you would dandelions, and eat it either raw in salads or cooked as greens. It is an excellent wild vegetable.

But if you would rather add it to your store of medicinal herbs, you will want not only the plant but its long roots, whose beneficial properties are especially high in spring and fall. Cut the roots up small and dry the rest of the plant in the usual fashion.

Pimpernel is an astringent plant that controls all sorts of hemorrhages, from nosebleeds to blood in the urine and abnormal vaginal bleeding. Its astringent powers extend to the intestinal tract as well—it halts diarrhea and dysentery.

In an emergency then, an infusion of pimpernel may stand you in good stead. For long-term use, prepare a decoction by boiling a handful of the plant, including a good bit of the root, in a quart of water for about ten minutes. Drink a wine glass of this several times a day.

This same mixture will check diarrhea.

Lavender

My mother's linen cupboard always smelled of lavender. I liked to watch her strew the little nodes of dried lavender between the freshly ironed sheets as she put them away. And when these heavy linen sheets were unfolded, they would be perfumed through and through with that clean bracing scent. To me lavender is always associated with good household linen resting in gleaming old armoires.

Some people also hang a bunch of lavender inside their clothes closet as protection against moths. Moths will indeed keep their distance from dried lavender.

Though lavender grows everywhere in Provence, there was little of it in the wooded country around Gavarret. However, my father knew where every tuft of it could be found. One day our dog Miss was bitten by a snake and my father set off at a run, heading for the nearest lavender patch about half a mile away. He was soon back, completely out of breath, and rubbed the puncture wound with the flowers. I was very upset and watched over Miss all night long, fearing for her life each time a spasm shook her fevered body. In the morning our dog was well again. Once more my father had performed what I considered a miracle.

In later years I have seen hunters in Provence gathering bunches of lavender precisely for the same purpose—for their hounds often blunder into poisonous snakes and are bitten. The antivenom action of lavender is well known in those parts.

Lavender can also be used as an antiseptic wash for wounds. Prepare a decoction by boiling a handful of lavender blossoms in a pint of water for ten minutes. Allow it to cool and apply it as a compress to the wound. The same preparation makes a healing lotion for eczemas, acne and burns. It may also be used as a douche against vaginal infections.

The strong scent of lavender, like mint, is a remedy for dizziness and fainting. Sometimes only dabbing the forehead and temples with lavender water will stave off a faint by stimulating the circulation to the brain. The same lavender water used as a rub on back and chest will clear congested air passages and quiet severe coughs. It is especially useful for whooping cough.

While lavender water is readily available commercially, you may enjoy making up your own supply. You simply steep 100 grams of lavender blossoms in a pint of alcohol for a few days. Keep the flask in a warm place where the temperature remains at about 90°F. Then strain and seal.

A few sprigs of lavender in the evening bath will calm the nerves and drive away germs. A lavender bath is most welcome in winter and helps throw off colds and flus. Boiling a few pinches of lavender and inhaling the vapor will also be beneficial in case of flu or bronchitis.

Gargling with lavender not only disinfects the throat, it can aid in overcoming certain speech defects such as stammering since the tranquilizing property of lavender relaxes the affected nerves and muscles. Lavender tea taken two or three times daily is exceedingly calming, almost sedative. It should therefore be used prudently. Nevertheless, in cases of severe headache, neuralgia, grippe, bronchitis, asthma or whooping cough, lavender tea is invaluable.

With all these uses for the herb, you will want to have a generous patch of lavender in your flower garden. The compact little bushes are a delight in themselves. Their bluish-violet flowers are as lovely as they are sweet-smelling, and while the plants are most at home in a warm climate, they withstand cold winters stoutly. If you live in the city and have no garden, look out for the lavender vendor who usually establishes herself close to the entrance of a major department store. You will know she is there before you see her, for her wicker basket is piled high with lavender sachets whose fragrance wafts far down the street. Buy a few sachets to put in your closets, and should you need some dried lavender in a hurry, you will only have to extract a packet or two from between the linens.

Couch Grass

No farmer will scold you if you trespass into his field to dig couch grass. For this is an invasive and stubborn weed and the bane of farmers. Nevertheless, the tenacity of certain plants is proof of their vigor: they possess powerful survival traits. Couch grass, for instance, develops an enormous root system that stretches in all directions. This is where the plant's strength is stored. Have you ever noticed how dogs and cats go into the fields in the spring and nibble on grass? It is couch grass they are eating. But to derive the fullest benefit from the plant, we should eat its roots. Pull up a clump of couch grass in the spring, wash the roots carefully, and cut them into small lengths for drying. They are even more effective in their fresh state.

These long fibrous roots of the couch grass used to be made into brooms. And, in fact, couch grass is a great cleanser. For a thorough spring-cleaning of your intestinal tract, make up a decoction of couch grass root. Since the root is rather tough and does not easily give up its juice, you will have to boil it at least ten minutes, whether fresh or dried. The taste will be improved by the addition of a little liquorice or lemon peel.

I remember an occasion when the proprietor of our one garage in Fleurance came to see my father. The man was suffering from kidney stone and was writhing in pain. The sight of such agony made a deep impression on my young mind. My father then and there had him drink a glass of couch grass and mint tea. We always had couch grass in the house; great bunches of the tangled roots were suspended from the rafters. Soon the man felt better. The pain eased and he managed to pass the stone. As it happened, the man's son was a schoolmate of mine and I heard from him that thereafter his father always drank a glass of couch grass and mint tea every morning, year in and year out, and his trouble never recurred.

I recommend this beverage for all ailments of the kidney and liver: jaundice, gallstones, bladder trouble, renal colic. It is also beneficial for gout and cellulite. For people in normal health, it makes an excellent diuretic and depurative.

Ivy

Because of its clinging and enfolding habits, ivy has become a metaphor for love and friendship. The ancients associated ivy with the close embrace of lovers. For the birds, ivy's dense evergreen foliage makes it an ideal refuge during the winter months when other trees are bare. They will nest in the thick cloak of ivy manteling walls and rocks, and certain species such as the ring dove will subsist upon the unripe fruit of the ivy. Other types of bird will wait until the spring and feed their nestlings with the now-ripened ivy berries. Bees, too, are well acquainted with the minute green flowers of the ivy, which are rich in nectar, and browse happily among ivy's leathery leaves.

Animals, on the other hand, have a somewhat guarded attitude toward ivy. Sheep and goats will sometimes nibble at it, for they have insatiable curiosity and iron stomachs. But domestic rabbits and dogs will have nothing to do with it: ivy contains hederin, which is toxic to certain animals. Cows, on the other hand, used to be given an armful of ivy to help them through difficult calvings.

Ivy's effect on man is twofold. It is somewhat dangerous for us, as it is for dogs. The fruits are especially so, and we should warn children not to taste the ivy berries. Yet in small amounts the leaves can be highly beneficial.

A tea of ivy leaves, highly diluted (a pinch of leaf to a quart of water) is an effective medicament against respiratory illnesses. It soothes coughs and helps clear mucous. Creeping ivy is best for such teas. Its leaves are more rounded than those of the climbing ivy. It carpets the woods and the edges of fields, especially in wet and shady spots. Pick it in the spring, when it comes into flower, gathering the green tips and drying them for use in the winter, when colds are frequent.

Some pharmaceutical houses have developed cough syrups based on ivy which are especially good for whooping cough. In olden days it was the custom to treat whooping cough by drinking wine that had been allowed to stand in a wooden goblet carved from the thick trunk of an ancient ivy vine. The ivy wood was supposed to transmit some of its virtues to the wine.

Like other bitter herbs, ivy stimulates the stomach and the digestive tract. It is also a diuretic.

But I treasure ivy most for its external uses. Above all, it can dissolve the lumps of fat associated with cellulite. Hence ivy is an ingredient in most anticellulite creams. I find I need great amounts of it and have my herb-gatherers collect all the creeping and climbing ivy for miles around. Dried ivy leaves take up many shelves in my herb house. Moreover, I am constantly renewing my supply, for ivy is available all year round. I use it in both creams and solutions.

You can easily prepare your own remedy for cellulite by making poultice of crushed ivy leaves and applying them to the affected areas. Another method is to boil ivy leaves for fifteen minutes in a quart of water and apply the solution in a wet dressing to the ugly puckerings. Complete the treatment by taking some herbal diuretic which rids your system of excess fluids, and you will soon see the cellulite disappear and your skin become firm and smooth again.

Ivy, which used to wreath the brows of poets, it now more apt to be bound around feminine contours. So in our day practical aims prevail. Yet we may still consider ivy to be associated with beauty, for is not the curve of a woman's thigh as lovely as any sonnet?

Mallow

Some flowers are gentle, others bitter and cruel. Mallow is surely one of the gentlest of blooms. Its artless blossoms are pale purple, the color of half-mourning, but in nature this color is not sorrowful in the least, but as rich with promise as spring itself.

Mallow is one of the ingredients of the "four-flower tea" which has been treasured over the centuries for its curative powers. To be accurate, this tea contains not four flowers but six: mallow, violet, poppy, mullein, colts foot and ground ivy—a piquant nosegay of field flowers to inspire the painter and poet. All these plants have tranquilizing powers.

Mallow is an emollient, that is to say it softens and soothes sensitive tissues. Its flowers and leaves make gargles and teas beneficial to the throat. In earlier days young children would be given the fibrous root of mallow to chew on while they were teething to cool their smarting gums. The mucilaginous juice extracted from mallow roots is used in certain throat lozenges.

The cultivated cousin of mallow is the hollyhock, whose tall spires give a picturesque, old-fashioned look to a garden. But the wild mallow is easily domesticated and looks particularly charming when combined with hollyhocks. Gather its leaves in the spring, its flowers in the summertime and its root in the fall. But you had best wait until the plant's second year to do this, when the root will have grown to some size. Dry the root and brush it carefully, but avoid washing it, for that might dilute the mucilaginous substance in which its virtue resides.

Wild mallow grows abundantly in the fields. In former times it was much favored for cooking and people would pick great basketfuls of the leaves for this purpose. It makes a delicate and bland soup, especially recommended for children and old people. Mallow leaves can also be used as greens, much like spinach. It is delicious when cooked with a mixture of other spring plants, such as borage, shepherd's purse, chickweed, plantain—all of which are soothing to the stomach and intestines.

The mildness of mallow makes it a particularly congenial herb for women. Either in the form of soup or teas, mallow can overcome stubborn constipation, otherwise so damaging to the figure and the complexion. A solution of mallow, used as a douche, will counter inflammation of the delicate female organs. The same solution makes an excellent facial lotion, dispersing blotches or skin irritations. As a mouthwash, it is effective against thrush.

All in all, mallow well deserves its Latin name of *althaea*, meaning comfort.

Poppy

The European wild poppy is closely related to the opium poppy and has similar properties. But let me quickly assure you that I am not going to tempt you into the type of drug abuse that has had such terrible effects on today's youth. The scarlet flower which brightens our wheat fields is far less dangerous than its oriental cousin.

Our field poppy, then, contains morphine but in extremely minute quantities. It is a tranquilizer but not a narcotic. Gather the petals of these lovely flowers, handling them gently, for they are as fragile as the most delicate silk. Spread them on paper and dry them in the open air, then store them in a closed jar.

If you have some doubts about a tea of pure poppy, you can use the petals along with linden blossoms, or as a component of the four-flower tea I mentioned earlier. These calming drinks are invaluable for treating sore throat, bronchitis, whooping cough, asthma and insomnia.

Shepherd's Purse

This plant takes its name from the shape of its seeds, which are flat and triangular and irresistibly suggestive of a purse, for it is also known as pastor's purse, capuchin's purse, Judas's purse or simply purselet.

It is a type of wild cress that grows all year round in milder climates. For medicinal purposes, the whole plant is picked (with the exception of the root), and dried or, even better, put through a juicer.

This is the most beneficial plant for all disorders of the blood. It checks hemorrhages, spitting of blood and nosebleeds. It tempers the sometimes excessive menstrual flow of girls at puberty and their mothers at the menopause. It helps against hemophilia. Both varicose veins and hemorrhoids show significant improvement after being treated with poultices of this plant applied to the congested areas.

A supply of shepherd's purse in dried form should be kept on hand for emergency use in household accidents.

Rose

When I begin speaking of roses, a sort of excitement grips me, for roses mean more to me than any other flower. When one falls in love, one ascribes to the loved person every desirable trait. So it is for me with roses, for I love them too well to take a detached view of them. A red rose is the very symbol of passion, glowing like desire itself. Yet because of the delicacy and softness of its petals it also calls to mind the soft cheeks of a girl and the exchange of innocent kisses. A whole romantic literature has grown up around the rose.

But let us be realistic. Apart from all these poetic associations, what can the rose do for us? To put it bluntly: can we eat it?

Goats do, but goats know no respect. For us to turn the rose to prosaic use may well be sacrilege.

There are, to be sure, all sorts of delicacies concocted from the rose: rose jelly, rose confections, rose honey, rose syrup, not to speak of rosewater, attar of roses and the like. The Arab countries have many sweets made with roses, and in the eighteenth century there was a rage for dousing everything with rosewater, from meats to sauces. But nowadays we value the rose only as a source of perfume, which is a pity.

For roses, and especially the red rose of Provence, have astringent and tonic properties that make them prime protection against diarrhea and dysentery. This would account for their popularity in hot climates where troubles of this sort are so prevalent. But roses are also effective against leukorrhea, tonsillitis and gingivitis. They lend themselves equally well to external and internal use. But, you will ask, in what form?

I am not going to ask you to denude your rose bushes. Let the buds unfold and take your joy of them, for surely that, too, contributes to your health. I do not cut my roses, either in my garden at Feucherolles near Paris or in my garden in the Gers. But as each blossom reaches its peak, just before it becomes overblown, I gather its petals. You can do likewise, and collect the velvety petals either to be dried for teas or to be used in their fresh state. Here is a simple recipe for a delicious spread that utilizes fresh rose petals:

Pound a quantity of rose petals with three times their weight in sugar. Add enough rosewater to give the mixture the consistency of honey. On bread or crackers, this is particularly favored by children.

My grandmother Sophie used to make a more elaborate form of rose jam. Since this was a luxury, I was allowed it only on Sundays. Grandmother once told me that my father had given her rose jam to General Pau, who was directing maneuvers in the neighborhood of Gavarret sometime in the years before World War I. The general had an atrocious cough, but our special rose jam made him well in a trice. The story made a strange impression on my childish mind and I nourished a grudge against this general for long afterward. Since Grandmother doled out her rose jam so parsimoniously, I thought it was because the general had eaten all of it. If it had not been for him, I might have had some every day.

You may make solutions of rose petals or add a few drops of commercial rosewater to other teas; the astringent property of the rose will act favorably on irritated intestines.

I have found that roses allay rheumatic pains. A handful of petals thrown into the bath will do wonders. The same discovery has been made by someone I know, a wealthy industrialist who shares my passion for the flower. He amused himself by throwing handfuls of rose petals from his garden into his bath from time to time and observed that he was no longer bothered by rheumatic aches. One day he mentioned the matter to me and I assured him that this was the effect of his roses.

You can prepare a rose vinegar (a handful of fresh rose petals steeped in vinegar) and use this as a rub. It cleanses the skin, acts as a disinfectant for pimples and sores and prevents their hurting.

May your life be as richly strewn with rose petals as is your garden and may you always have roses about you, both in your preserve cupboard and on your dressing table. For roses are a pledge of health and beauty.

Violet

My father used to smell of violets. It was his favorite scent and he would prepare it himself for his own use. But in this taste he had a famous predecessor. Vulcan, the blacksmith god, once came to pay court to Venus all perfumed with violets and made such a favorable impression on her that the goddess, who had previously repulsed him, gave him a kiss.

As a matter of fact, violets are suggestive of kisses. They are the most tender of flowers, with the most elusive of fragrances. They are good against coughs and loss of voice. I always recommend violets to singers who come to me to learn how to protect their precious vocal chords from cold and germs. It is not merely out of local pride that I recommend candied violets, a speciality of Toulouse and thus a product of my home region. In earlier times people would make all sorts of confections from violets:

jams and flower pastes, as well as the violet syrup which was considered a household necessity to be kept for use in the winter. Here is the recipe:

Gather a pound of fresh violets. Put them in a large kettle and add two quarts of boiling water. Let them steep for half a day, keeping the mixture warm, either on the back of the stove or on a radiator. Strain and add two pounds of sugar. Let this simmer for an hour or two in a double doiler, then pour into jars and seal.

Such violet syrup can be used either as a gargle or as a delicious tea. Two or three spoonfuls are enough for a cup. It is the gentlest remedy for sore throats, colds, bronchitis, whooping cough and asthma. You can also brew a tea from plain violets, allowing about twelve blossoms to a cup, which will have the same pacifying qualities.

Violet leaves are mildly laxative. They should be picked in the spring before the flowers come, and dried. A tea of violet leaves and flowers will have the combined virtues of both and will benefit both the digestive functions and the respiratory tract.

As for the root, it has a stronger action than the rest of the plant. It is a purgative and an emetic. If you should have a bout of indigestion or a touch of food poisoning, drink a decoction of violet root to clean out your stomach. To make this decoction, boil 15 grams of violet root for ten minutes. The roots should first be chopped fine, for they are very dense.

Nasturtium

It has the reputation of arousing sexual appetites, and hence is sometimes called "love-flower." Though nasturtium originated in Peru, it is now a favorite the world over. Its piquant blossoms in every hue ranging from the palest yellow to burning scarlet, its neat round leaves and rollicking habit of growth, and its easy culture should earn it a place in even the smallest garden.

The leaves make a good addition to a potato soup. The flowers may be eaten in a salad, while also adding a flash of color. The still-green seeds may be pickled in vinegar and served as capers.

All parts of the plant, except for the root, have a peppery taste that is stimulating to the appetite and this may be the preface to other desires and pleasures with which the nasturtium is associated.

With its high sulphur content, nasturium is especially good for older people and greatly increases their energy. Its gently laxative quality has a beneficial effect on the digestion.

Used externally, nasturtium has long been known as a remedy against baldness. Hence it is an ingredient in many hair tonics. Here is a tried-and-true recipe for such a compound: gather 100 grams of nasturtium leaves, along with the same quantity of box foliage and nettles. Steep these in a quart of alcohol for two weeks, keeping the mixture at 90°F. Strain and bottle. Rub well into the scalp. Keep this up faithfully and before too long the bare spots will be covered by a splendid new crop of hair, thanks to the nasturtium.

Hawthorn

In France the hawthorn grows in every hedgerow. My father used to go out in the lovely month of May and gather baskets of the tiny white hawthorn blossoms, which my mother would then carefully dry. So it pains me that the hawthorn is disappearing from the land, as hedgerows are eliminated in favor of larger fields fenced with barbed wire. One of these days there will be no hedgerows left and where will we find hawthorn?—a flower close to my heart and rightly so, for it has a direct bearing on that organ.

Hawthorn blossoms are a valuable remedy against cardiac and nervous disorders. They do wonders for insomnia, palpitations of the heart, angina, hypertension and similar grave problems. A tea of hawthorn blossoms relaxes overwrought nerves and summons peaceful sleep. Hence the slander that hawthorn blossoms repress sexual desire. But then, that is a common charge against the tranquilizing herbs.

The virtues of the blossoms are well known and recognized by the medical profession. In Germany the pharmacies carry an extract of hawthorn that is specifically prescribed for angina pectoris. As for the dried blossoms, they are available wherever herbal products are for sale.

My father was often consulted about heart irregularities. He would go about calming the heart by applying a wet dressing of hawthorn blossoms and this would often have the desired effect. No wonder my father had the greatest faith in the power of these dainty flowers.

Borage

Borage could say, and it would be true,
I comfort the heart, I banish all rue.

Again, a mnemonic verse from the medical school of Salerno. I cannot personally vouch for its claims. While the ancients held that borage could banish melancholy, my own experience indicates that it can overcome malignant fevers—in thus restoring people to health it would also, naturally, restore their smiles.

A familiar potherb, with its sky-blue flowers and furry leaves, borage deserves a place in the flower garden. It should also be considered for culinary purposes, for its leaves make delectable greens and its flowers add a fresh taste, much like cucumbers, to any salad.

Leaves and flowers should also be dried and kept on hand as a weapon against sudden fevers due to measles, scarlet fever, bronchitis or flu. Borage also brings relief from rheumatism. A borage tea containing both flowers and leaves reduces fever and is a welcome soprific.

The juice of fresh borage, gathered in the spring, makes an excellent depurative. A tiny glass of it, taken at breakfast, will thoroughly rejuvenate the kidneys.

Yarrow

Achilles used this plant to treat his wounds, hence its botanical name: achillea. It also has a host of folk names—woundwort, carpenter's grass, butcherswort and soldierswort—all linking it to occupations highly prone to cuts or gashes. It would seem that the efficacy of yarrow has long been known.

The juice of yarrow, applied to a cut or a gash, will stop bleeding and speed the healing process.

A solution of yarrow leaves has the same astringent properties. It arrests hemorrhages, relieves painful menstruation, soothes hemorrhoids and dispels congestion in all the organs.

It is one of the most common wild flowers, growing in meadows, pastures and along roadsides. Its pungent foliage should be part of every household store of useful herbs.

Cow-Parsnip

Its old name was poor-man's beer, for an alcoholic drink can be made from it. The flowers and leaves are stripped off and only the stem is utilized. This is boiled in water and allowed to steep for a few days. After being fermented, the drink is somewhat like beer.

The stems of cow-parsnip have a high sugar content. Set to dry in the sun, the stems will exude droplets of a honeylike juice much enjoyed by children.

The leaves make a good vegetable, especially added to soup. Some have maintained that the famous borscht of the Russians is really based on cow-parsnip, the other vegetables, such as beets and cabbage, being mere supplements. Like mallow and borage, cow-parsnip is an emollient and acts as a balm to the stomach and intestines.

As with all the umbelliferae, such as the wild carrot and caraway, the lacy flower of the cow-parsnip ripens into a circlet of tasty seeds. These are supposed to have aphrodisiac qualities. A tea is made from them. My father used to include these seeds in several of his preparations, and was inclined to classify the cow-parsnip as one of the herbs of happiness.

Corn Silk

We all know what substantial food value is packed into an ear of corn. But for my special purposes I am more interested in the corn silk, that skein of golden threads found immediately under the papery corn husk. I gather it before the silk begins to brown and when the ear of corn is still largely unformed.

Dried in the sun, corn silk is one of the most dependable of diuretics. Potent though it is, it has no bad side effects and is thus suitable for chronic illnesses that require prolonged treatment, perhaps continuing for several weeks.

A tea made from this corn silk taken faithfully every day will offset the retention of urine and help dissolve bladder stones. It is also good against stubborn cases of cystitis and renal colic. Last but not least, it helps against rheumatism.

5. Sickness: An Alarm Signal

*Nature is the best doctor of all, for she cures
three-quarters of our sicknesses, and what is more,
she never speaks ill of other doctors.*

The remark is Galen's, whose treatises on medicine, written in
the second century, laid the basis for medical science. Galen was
a wise and humorous observer of the human condition and the
forgoing aphorism is as true as ever. Doctors are often astonished
when a patient whom they have given up for lost suddenly and
for no apparent reason recovers. What has happened is that nature has taken charge of the case. The wisest doctors will concede
nature her part and will recognize her stamp and pay homage to
her feats.

Mental illnesses may be especially susceptible to natural cures.
According to the newest school of psychiatry—which takes a vir-
tually antipsychiatric line—some of the most serious forms of
mental derangement would in time resolve themselves if the person were not subjected to brutal mistreatment.

We must be careful, however, not to mistake this doctrine for
a dangerous form of neglect and inertia. I am all for welcoming
nature's help, but I am also for mobilizing all the means at our
command for meeting her halfway.

When an illness strikes us—and illness does strike, there is no
denying that—we must not sit by with folded arms, leaving the
issue to nature. On the contrary, we must analyze the character
of the illness, for unless we know that we may resort to quite the
wrong measures, which will hinder rather than help the body find
its way back to proper functioning. Have you ever seen a man
swim against the current? He wastes his strength in futile floun-

derings and soon gives up entirely. But it is quite different
with the swimmer who swims with the current. His body stretches
close to the water's surface. He lets the current carry him along
and the pull of the water makes each of his strokes count for double. Soon he steps out fresh and vigorous on a welcoming shore.

It is the same with our health. The rude blows that interrupt
the course of our lives should be understood as alarms. Something
is not right about the way we are living. We have in some way
gone off the track. We must try to restore the vital current again.
We must muster our inner forces, reform our habits and reshape
our patterns. We must reach out toward what is good and cheering
and strengthening, to what nourishes body and soul and is as
sustaining as the kisses of our children.

When sickness strikes, bring all your arms to bear against it.
Gather your personal riches and hold them fast in your embrace.
Avail yourself of every helpful factor: a good bed, certainly, but
also good reading, good music, a rose at the bedside table, a
steaming glass of herbal tea whose blessings you believe in and
a loving person to prepare and serve it. Your trusted family doctor
plays an important role. He knows your physical state better than
anyone else. He is almost a friend, and will know how to guide
you toward restored health, leading you by the hand and setting
the pace of your progress. The best doctor is a prudent one
who will not do violence to your nature by hurrying you along
too fast, but will rather slow you down so that your recovery is
deep and thorough.

I have always worked in collaboration with medical men, and
I ask my patients to bring me an authorization from their doctor.
I have thus received hundreds, even thousands, of testimonials of
confidence. And I reciprocate this confidence. My best results
have always been obtained by working in concert with a doctor.
When medical measures failed to give the patient the strength
to throw off the illness, my modest collaborative treatment often
provided the necessary impetus.

But I do not harbor any illusions about my own powers. Some
of the credit belongs to the patient himself and his will to recover.
Some of the credit belongs to his family and their willingness to
cooperate with me. Some of the credit belongs to the doctor,
whose diagnosis is based on long experience. Only then do I come

in, with my packets of herbs, which represent messages of hope from nature. And if my role were only to lead the patient back to the path of health, that would be quite enough and I would not want to claim that I had done more. One of my American patients, a banker, sometimes calls me from New York to ask advice. I cured him of chronic asthma and he has the highest opinion of my powers. He has since taken up singing in a serious way and wants to become a concert artist. But of course, my plants cannot help him there and I try to make him understand that I am no wonder-worker in this sense.

To my way of thinking, a person who has dedicated his life to the service of others, whether as doctor or plant-healer, must know his limits. Confucius, whose wisdom consisted in accepting the human condition with humility, said: To know what one knows and to know what one does not know, that is true knowledge. Thus the good doctor is one who does not sin either in the direction of vanity or timidity.

I try to adhere to this principle. There are illnesses I cannot treat and I have always firmly refused to try to. Many times people have come to me in a desperate state of mind begging me to do something for them. But the best service I could do them was to declare my powerlessness and send them away empty-handed. This is always very difficult in human terms, but I feel strongly that one must not deceive people or lull them with false promises. Instead, I try to direct people to the specialist or surgeon whom they ought to see.

If, on the other hand, I encounter someone with an ailment I have often dealt with, where I am confident of positive results, I take over without reservations: I make the patient's cause my own and I stake my pride on effecting a cure, since I know that my plants will do the trick. To be sure, I have had failures, for some cases are highly complex or extremely advanced. But I aim for the smallest risk. My personal records (which I have always kept day by day, despite my dislike for figures, because they provide me with moral support) have always been immensely useful in this regard.

For twenty-five years now I have refused to treat cancer. Here is a realm where neither my plants nor I make any claim. Now that I am in my fifties I am more and more concerned with the philosophical aspect of things. I have learned a great deal, listened, thought, and thus extended the scope of my science without changing its base. I am more and more concerned with long-term solutions. I no longer take individual cases, not only because of the pressures of time but also because my long involvement with lawsuits has shown me that one can go on indefinitely wasting one's strength crossing swords with scattered but implacable enemies. Instead, I try to do something for people at large and use my talents to attack those social problems that are intimately bound up with public health.

By now it is fairly well established that certain conditions are cancer-inducing: air and water pollution, chemical additives in food, the habit of smoking, faulty hygiene. I have decided that I want to use my energies to fight this scourge at its source, since once it is diagnosed in a person I am powerless against it. Health consists of making of one's body a strong and fruitful plot of ground, productive of the good and impregnable to infection. I speak of "ground" because I am basically a gardener, with human nature as my garden.

So I shall spend my life from now on sowing, hoeing, watering and raking. And if, at fifty, I no longer go through my garden every morning picking off the aphids, it is because I trust things to come through such minor troubles. I prefer to prepare the soil so well that the plants can withstand a few insects. I feel the same way about my sons as they grow up. I no longer have to stand by to pick them up when they tumble. They have learned to walk, to negotiate the rough spots in the road. I am still guiding them, I hope, but from a distance.

We must each of us, then, learn to live with the constitutions which are ours by birth, for good or ill, and present a mixture of strengths and weaknesses. In antiquity, Hippocrates informs us, people were classified according to their temperaments. There were four categories: the sanguine, the nervous, the bilious and the lymphatic, each group requiring different treatment. Though this classification of human types is excessively schematic, there is much good sense in the idea. Today we would greatly multiply the categories and incorporate considerations of heredity, environment and climate. But the truth remains that everyone must work out his own particular pattern in order to live in harmony with his body.

My recommendations, then, are meant in a general sense. I never treated a sickness, but a sick person. Nowadays I no longer attack specific ailments but attempt to arm people against the perils to our health arising from the changing conditions of life. Yet it is hard to generalize about these matters and I want to keep my teachings flexible so that each individual may draw upon them to develop sane and practicable rules adapted to his own needs.

My experience has been largely based on chronic ailments or long-term problems. In emergency cases I would have been called in too late, for my treatments by their very nature must operate over a longer time span. I do think I have given my patients a renewed joy in life, so necessary for getting well, and they have aided me immeasurably by their patience. The following section then, is written with this principle in mind. To the man crippled by acute articular rheumatism, I say: "You must see a doctor immediately." But to someone who is periodically visited by an old rheumatic condition, I say: "My friend, let us go over your mode of life together and discover what mistakes have brought you to this pass. Then I will show you how to retrace your steps and right your inner balance." And with faith, the patient will presently see his trouble gradually abate.

I want also to stress that my treatments and prescriptions are meant to be followed carefully. I have mentioned one case where a patient overlooked my directions and used the herbs I had sent to make a tea when I had intended them for a foot bath. But quite apart from such comical accidents, many people go about preparing the herbs in a haphazard way, when exactitude is necessary. Let me then review the terms most often used in these prescriptions and make sure that they are properly understood.

There are several ways to extract the active principle from plants. The most common method is *infusion*. This consists of pouring boiling water over the leaves or flowers, either fresh or dried, and letting the mixture steep for a few minutes, covered, while the plant's juices pass into the water. This method is the preferred way of dealing with delicate herbs such as mint, linden, verbena, and flowers such as camomile, violet and orange blossom.

Another method is *decoction*, which is reserved for plants of tougher substance, for thick coarse leaves, roots and seeds—whether fresh or dry. Material of this sort has to be boiled in water for several minutes, ten minutes usually being the maximum.

Maceration involves soaking the plant material in a liquid, usually at room temperature. The liquid is not necessarily water; it is more likely wine, vinegar or oil. The process is a slow one, requiring weeks or even months, as when aromatic herbs are steeped in vinegar.

Some of these preparations are taken as a *tisane*, that is, as a tea, which may or may not be sugared. On the whole it is best not to sugar them; honey may be used for sweetening. I do not think it necessary to give exact measurements for most of these tisanes. Usually you will want a pinch of the dried plant to a cup of water. The pinch corresponds to 4 or 5 grams of the plant when fresh. Sometimes I call for a smaller pinch or a larger pinch, according to the potency of the herb. Mixed tisanes, which include a combination of herbs, are best made up in larger batches, using, say, a quart of water, and drunk several times in the course of the day, reheating a cup at a time. Where four or five herbs are called for, it becomes difficult to measure a pinch which will represent the various plants in equal proportion.

These three types of preparation—infusion, decoction and maceration—are not always for drinking purposes. They may be used as gargling solutions, mouthwashes, antiseptic solutions, vaginal douches, wet dressings, etc.

In my own practice I have often used these preparations for hand and foot baths. From earliest times medicine has relied on the principle of osmosis. The hands and feet are the most absorbant areas of the body. Doctors and scientists corroborate me in this. Here, for example, is an excerpt from a letter to me by Mr. L. R., a noted botanist who was for a long time director of Botanical Studies at the Colonial Institute in Marseilles:

> I turn to you because I am convinced that the potent substances of plants, extracted by maceration, can more effectively be introduced into the body through the epidermis than by oral ingestion or intravenous injection.
>
> I have personal knowledge of a good many instances where typhoid fever, malaria and other tropical diseases were quickly overcome when certain plants were crushed and bound around the sick person's wrists.

Yet precisely because these treatments by osmosis are extremely powerful, I would advise the utmost caution in their use. My prescriptions for hand and foot baths include certain herbs in homeopathic doses, for their action is otherwise too drastic. People without experience in this field should not attempt such therapy. On the other hand, the recipes I give for food, teas and other external treatments are easy to follow and involve no risk. Whenever a plant presents some counter indication or danger, I call attention to the fact. Thus camomile in massive doses will produce vomiting, celandine is toxic, marjoram is stupefying and sage can cause hypertension.

The list of illnesses I discuss in the following section is not, of course, exhaustive. My approach is to group these illnesses under the heading of the organ directly involved: the liver, the respiratory system, the intestines, the heart, etc. I have also given priority to those illnesses I have successfully treated and know to be susceptible to cure by plants. I have said nothing about those grave diseases that are beyond my scope, such as cancer, heart disease and tuberculosis. These require swift medical attention.

The Liver

It should be obvious that there is a direct relationship between the state of the liver and diet. Some people suffer from liver deficiency and must be careful all their lives to eat in such a way as not to overtax this organ. People who have been suddenly stricken by a liver attack must learn to follow a strict regimen, for that is their first step toward recovery.

While rich food, fatty meats, sauces, fried dishes, starches, pastries and alcohol are the sworn enemies of the liver, most green vegetable and fruits are the liver's friends. When the liver gives trouble, you can do no better than to go on a vegetarian diet. The benefits from this will be manifold.

However, there are certain vegetables that have to be avoided. On the proscribed list are members of the cabbage family (red cabbage, brussels sprout, cauliflower, broccoli), some root vegetables such as turnip and celery root, as well as spinach and cucumbers. Among the fruits you had better stay away from are banana, melons, apricots and prunes. Finally, raw foods tend to be hard to digest. You will do better to rely on soups, boiled vegetables and compotes.

A number of vegetables act on the irritated liver like medicines. The foremost among these are dandelion and artichoke. When I was a boy neighbors would often come to consult Father because someone in their family was down with jaundice. And Father, I remember, would always advise that the patient be given dandelions and artichokes, in every form, raw and cooked, in salads and in soups. He would offer the people a great stalk of artichoke from our own garden, or else the dried leaves of artichoke from his stores. He would explain how a tisane should be made from these portions of the artichoke and suggest that the tea be mixed with tea made from dandelion.

"The root of the dandelion should also go into it," he would say. "The bitterer the brew is, the sooner you'll be well."

It has been established that eating dandelion doubles the secretion of bile within half an hour.

Among the other vegetables that benefit the liver are carrot, watercress, all the salad greens (which should perhaps be eaten braised), tomato and olive. With regard to the olive, there is a simple and efficacious remedy I have always prescribed for people with liver complaints: Every morning before breakfast take a tablespoon of pure high-quality olive oil. If this seems rather nasty on an empty stomach, add a few drops of lemon juice or else eat a slice of lemon with it. The olive oil awakens and stimulates a lazy gallbladder or a distressed liver. During periods of liver trouble you should use no other seasonings but olive oil and lemon, adding perhaps garlic if it does not disagree with you.

Along with lemon, the other citrus fruits have a benign effect on the liver: oranges, tangerines and grapefruits help keep the liver in balance. Grapes are also highly recommended for their depurative action, and apples, the finest fruit of all, soothe and regulate.

As the symptoms of liver malfunction abate, you can gradually return to a more varied diet. Begin by eating small amounts of lean meat, fish and dairy products—preferably those made from skimmed milk.

You have to give up all forms of alcohol, coffee and carbonated beverages during your illness, but do not reduce your fluid intake. In fact, you need to drink more than usual to help rid your system of toxic substances. Mineral water is usually recommended, and there are some brands specifically intended for liver complaints. You will also derive great benefits from tisanes. You may not have access to artichoke leaves or dandelion roots, but teas made of sage, rosemary and mint are also beneficial to the liver.

If you are prone to liver upsets, I would advise you to keep a stock of the most useful plants on hand and turn to them at the first signs of trouble. You might also cultivate the habit of drinking the following tea as a preventive measure, for it is a veritable balm to the sensitive liver. For a day's supply (four cups) you will want a quart of water and a pinch of the following herbs: sage flowers, rhubarb root, pimpernel (the entire plant is used), dandelion (the entire plant) and Great Centaury. If for some reason you cannot make up the mixture, the separate plants are equally good.

If you are suffering severe pain on the right side, you can obtain relief by applying hot compresses to the place. For additional help, soak the compress in a solution of the herbs previously cited. Another method for dealing with the pain of a liver attack is to apply a poultice made from chopped cabbage and chopped watercress moistened with beaten egg white.

To conclude: It is well to know that liver attacks are often psychological in origin, arising from frustrations, nervous shocks and so forth. You should therefore consider what you can do to remove the causes. Allow yourself more rest, improve the quality of your sleep and attempt to put your life, at least physically, on a sounder basis. Anything that contributes to this aim is good: daily exercise, fresh air, a better work schedule, good rest and regular meals.

Thus, in ministering to your liver, you will be doing good to your whole self.

The Stomach

The stomach is prone to a great many ills, all the way from lack of appetite to ulcers. Some of them are mild and passing indispositions, others are serious and call for the attention of a doctor. Many of these troubles are of nervous origin. Thus cramps and acidity are the result of eating too fast in an atmosphere of tension. And as we all know, the success-seeker is more subject to ulcers than he who is less concerned with this sort of achievement.

The first rule for dealing with an ailing stomach is to eliminate obvious sources of nervous tension. The second is to banish all acid, sharp foods and irritants from your diet. This means tart fruits and fruit juices, raw vegetables, vinegar, spices, alcohol, coffee, carbonated drinks and tobacco. Choose foods that are mild in taste and soft in texture. If, on the other hand, your stomach is languid and your appetite at a low ebb, you may enliven your interest in food by such garnishes as black radish (be careful of this at first) and seasonings such as tarragon, sage and basil. These add piquancy to any dish, from eggs to salads and soups.

Should cramps and acidity persist even after you have modified your diet, try the various tisanes that are calming to the stomach such as camomile, mint, savory and verbena. You might also try the celebrated melissa cordial, which goes back to the Middle Ages when the monks of the Carmelite order created this aromatic liqueur that has ever since been known as a remarkable tonic for tempermental digestions. Its chief ingredient is the herb melissa, and this may be used in infusions like any other herb. Let me also suggest a mixed tisane consisting of two pinches of basil (the entire plant), one pinch of camomile blossom and one pinch of peppermint steeped in a quart of boiling water. Take four cups of this in the course of the day.

If you are bothered by wind, you will be benefited by the so-called carminative herbs: angelica, anise, cumin, caraway and fennel. Eat the fennel either raw or boiled, the angelica candied or in a compote of stewed fruits, and the caraway seed in bread or cake. Anise and cumin are generally used as spices but the seeds may also be used for tisane. There is also the old-fashioned "four-seed tea," which is at once delicious and curative. It consists of equal parts of anise seed, fennel seed, caraway and coriander.

Should you feel a spell of indigestion coming on and have no medicinal herbs on hand, remember the parsley tea my grandmother used to serve after a heavy meal, always to such good effect.

Finally, if by mischance you have eaten something toxic or spoiled and your stomach balks at receiving it, help your stomach right itself. If you haven't the courage to thrust two fingers down your throat, make up an emetic drink. This may be a very heavy infusion of camomile (the usual mild infusion of one pinch to a cup has a calming effect, so you had better quadruple the doses) or a decoction of violet root (two or three pinches of the chopped up root, boiled for ten minutes in a cup of water).

A grumbling stomach may be quieted by applying a warm compress or a hot-water bottle to it after a meal. I imagine everyone knows where his stomach is located. Concerning the other organs, people's notions are somewhat less precise—most of us seem quite vague about anatomy.

The Intestines

There are people who seem condemned to veer between constipation and colic and never to know normal intestinal functioning. The usual reason is that they have destroyed the balance and the rhythm of their body by the abuse of medicaments. Having first taken an overdose of some strong laxative to overcome their constipation, they find that their irritated intestines will not behave. They must therefore control their disturbing diarrhea by astringent medicine, which tightens their bowels again. And so it goes.

The medicinal plants are far less concentrated than these medicaments and affect the body in a gentler, more gradual way. So if you suffer from chronic constipation, do not resort to the drastic commercial laxatives but instead give a large place in your diet to fruits and vegetables, whether raw or cooked, with special emphasis on spinach, fennel, all the greens. Vegetable soups will be particularly helpful.

On the other hand, canned goods, spices and commercially prepared foods high in sugar and preservatives will be bad for you. You can easily dispense with these non-nutritious products, and will be all the better for it. Here is an opportunity to learn new health habits. For breakfast have some good whole-grain bread with honey and a dish of stewed prunes. Like people with liver trouble, make a practice of having a tablespoon of olive oil every morning. Avail yourself of lots of rhubarb, stewed or in pies, as a jam or a tea. And in the fall embark on a grape cure, which will cleanse your system of all impurities and leave your intestines in fine working order.

Allow yourself a morning cigarette. Why not? Many people feel that a cigarette is necessary to ease their morning bowel movement and I would not be so stern as to deny it to them. But I would also urge them to do some setting up exercises, with special attention to those that strengthen the abdominal region. Here is a prime way to tone up those lazy intestinal muscles. If you cannot set aside five minutes in the morning for gymnastics, find occasions in the course of the day—when, for instance, you are alone in the elevator, or in similar empty and private moments, to tighten and relax your stomach muscles a dozen times or so as you stand. This in itself constitutes an excellent workout for the intestinal muscles.

If you would like a helpful tea, I recommend one made with a pinch of mallow blossom, two pinches of rosemary blossom and four pinches of wild chicory leaf steeped in a quart of water. Drink two cups of this in the course of the day.

Napoleon made use of a purgative created for him by his personal physician, Dr. Larrey, and known as the "emperor's lemonade." Here is the recipe: Slice three lemons and combine with 24 grams of senna. Steep for twenty-four hours in three cups of water. Add 60 grams of sugar and drink this mixture three times in the course of the day. Napoleon, an early riser, would have his first glass at six in the morning, his second at eight and his third glass at one in the afternoon. You will perhaps want to move the hours up a bit.

Diarrhea can be an even more serious problem. Young children in particular can be rapidly weakened by a bout of this. They should immediately be put on a diet of carrots, either strained or as a soup. The doctor should be consulted without delay.

An adult has greater reserves and is not in any danger unless the diarrhea is acute and prolonged. It may be a dysentery caused by a virus of some sort, requiring strong measures; or it may be a passing condition that will straighten out with the proper dietary adjustmets. Boiled rice is the tried-and-true remedy. To be most effective, the rice should retain all its starch. This means it should not be washed or rinsed but allowed to cook into a sticky mass, which may not be the preferred way to eat it but is best for the purpose. You should also avoid those fruits and vegetables that are recommended for constipation.

Your stock of preserves can serve as excellent medicines for these everyday ailments if you know the different properties of your jams and jellies. Just as you reach for prune and rhubarb jams as first-aid against constipation, you should resort to quince and blueberry jellies to alleviate diarrhea. A few spoonfuls of either of these on top of your bowl of rice makes a tasty dessert and will settle your bowels in short order.

A tisane of nettles or of pimpernel will alleviate diarrhea or colic. Pimpernel can also be used as a wash to soothe irritated tissues in case of prolonged dysentery. Fifty grams of the plant should be boiled in a quart of water for fifteen minutes.

I also recommend a simple and soothing tisane made with a pinch of peppermint blossom and two pinches of angelica root to a quart of water. Two glasses of this per day will bring comfort to the ravaged intestines.

In case of colon bacillus infection, here is a most soothing infusion: two pinches of heather blossom and two of fragrant woodruff (the entire plant is used) in a quart of water. Have four cups of this in the course of the day.

The intestines sometimes fall prey to worms, either a single tapeworm or a host of small intestinal parasites that are difficult to dislodge. The best weapon against these is garlic in all its forms—raw, cooked or worn as an amulet about the neck. There are other milder vermifuges—pumpkin, squash, carrot and thyme are all effective.

The Kidneys and Bladder

I recall that one of my patients once came to me with her dog and begged me to do something for the poor animal. She had gone to a number of vets, all of whom had given up on the case.

The poor beast suffered from cystitis—there was blood in its urine and it was evidently in perpetual discomfort. I prescribed a tea of sage and mallow, to be mixed with the animal's food. In only a few days I heard that the animal's urine had become clear again. But its devoted mistress went on giving her dog a tisane of mallow and sage for the remainder of its days in order to prevent any relapses.

Such quick results are always gratifying and can often be obtained with animals and children, whose bodies are less clogged with chemical products than those of adults. In pursuit of health, many people try this or that treatment in a confused fashion and end by well-nigh poisoning themselves. Dogs and children react more directly and sensitively, which is why I am always careful to prescribe only the lightest doses for them.

One can often clean up health problems in a child without having recourse to any medicines. Sometimes a small child will have difficulty with its urine because of some muscular contraction in the urinary tract. In a case of this sort one need only open a faucet near the child. The sound of running water will, by conditioned reflex, unblock the bladder. Conversely, children who have trouble with urinary control will often wet themselves at the mere sound of running water.

Adults are less susceptible to such simple suggestion. Yet it is worthwhile trying such tricks in conjunction with more substantial treatment.

Any difficulty in urinating must be dealt with quickly, for the retention of urine may lead to a poisoning of the total organism. The chlorates, sugars and uric acid carried in the urine must be quickly voided or they will lead to serious illness such as uremia, gout, albuminaria, diabetes and edema.

There are many natural diuretics that encourage healthy urination without resort to medicines. Everyone can decide which one he prefers and vary his choice according to the season and his other health considerations. To some people I will recommend a good dish of strawberries every evening during the strawberry season. Not only is this a delectable dessert, but a strawberry cure refreshes the entire body. To a somewhat fastidious city man I will say: "Drink a cup of cherry stem tea every evening. The product is available at any health food shop." To a farmer, who has fields of corn at his disposal, I will say: "Take some corn silk and make a tisane of it. A glass of this every evening will soon put you to rights." To a heavy eater I will say: "Include lots of onions in your meals." If, moreover, I want to chastise him somewhat (for his heavy eating is doing him no good), I will recommend that he treat himself with onion wine. Here is the recipe: Take 250 grams of onions and chop them fine. Mix with 100 grams of honey and a pint of white wine. The mixture is curious-tasting but effective. Three or four spoonfuls should be taken daily.

As a general rule, green vegetables, fruits and herbal teas of various kinds all have diuretic properties. They are the cleansers of the bladder and should be constants in your diet. If the body shows a tendency to retain urine or fluids, you should cut down on salt and spices and avail yourself of the more powerful plant diuretics. These are dandelion, either raw in salad or boiled or as a tea (the root should be included); couch grass root as a tea; borage and mallow, which you may have in the form of soups if you prefer them that way; and the choicest leaves from your strawberry bed or raspberry row, which make delicate tisanes.

Should your albumen count be high, add a pinch of juniper needles to a quart of your dandelion tea.

If your condition is more serious and the urinary tract seems highly inflamed, with danger of cystitis or prostate difficulties, you should try heather, which, like the sage I recommended in the case of the dog, is at once soothing and antiseptic. You will want to prepare a strong decoction of heather blossoms—two pinches boiled in a quart of water for fifteen minutes. Continue to boil the mixture with the cover off until the water is reduced by half. Drink two or three cups of this during the day.

The problem of urinary incontinence usually troubles old people or children, but it may also afflict pregnant women or women in menopause. My recommendation is to soak in a hip bath prepared in the following fashion: Bring three quarts of water to the boiling point. Add a good-sized garlic bulb, well chopped, a handful of hawthorn blossoms and another handful of buttercups (both flowers and leaves). Let the mixture steep for four or five hours. Strain it and store the liquid in a glass or china vessel. This quantity will do for several hip baths. Make sure you warm the mixture before adding it to the bath so that you do not lower the temperature of the bath water, which should be as hot as you can tolerate.

Rheumatism

When winter rolls around, all sorts of miseries commence. And when our lives reach their winter phase, these miseries often settle into our weary old bones.

No one dies of rheumatism; in fact, people who have it may live to the ripest old age. But they are often in great pain. Medicine is for the most part powerless to cure rheumatism. At most, it offers some relief during the worst phase of a crisis—until the next onslaught.

Rheumatism, gout and arthritis are all different manifestations of the same illness—a blockage in a joint, whether it be the knee, shoulder, hip, wrist, fingers or big toe. However, there are a wide variety of causes. Some people are arthritic by temperment, predisposed from an early age to weakness in their joints. Heredity is a considerable factor. Heavy eaters, who never knew these ills in their earlier years, with age must suddenly pay the penalty for their alimentary excesses: uric acid collects in their joints and causes inflammation and they come down with gout.

Accidents can also bring on rheumatism—either some sort of jolt or fracture that leaves the joints particularly vulnerable, or a virus that enters the body in the wake of a flu. Illnesses such as angina or gonorrhea that have not received proper treatment may infect the cartilaginous tissue. With any attack of rheumatic fever, a doctor should be consulted without delay, for there is the danger of cardiac complications.

In case of gout it goes without saying that the patient must change his eating habits. He must keep to an austere diet, avoiding all fatty meats, game, fried foods, starches, pastries, spices, alcohol and coffee. In addition, people prone to gout should exercise strenuously in order to burn up the toxins that will otherwise accumulate in their joints. Unfortunately people with gout are apt to be physically lazy as well as gluttonous. They should be made to realize that they themselves must take responsibility for getting well.

If rheumatism arises from accidental causes, an austere diet is still indicated in order to subdue the inflammation. The previous list of forbidden foods must be widened to include foods that aggravate the decalcification of the bones: vinegar, spinach, pickles, rhubarb, apricots, tomatoes. On the other hand, one should include all the dairy foods in one's diet, for they are rich in calcium and help strengthen the bones. Cabbage is also very good, and onions, cress, thyme, parsley and currents.

Besides diet and exercise, there are some thermal cures that can be extremely helpful to a chronic condition. But warmth is always the best remedy. People with rheumatism do well to flee cold climates and seek out lands of sunshine. But since this is not always possible, they should take every advantage of what sources of warmth there are at home. In my native Gascony where the sun shines generously, the old folk always have a bench against the house wall where they install themselves in the springtime, as soon as the sunlight has some strength to it. As they put it, they are "warming their aches and pains."

I would recommend to people with rheumatism that they always keep the sensitive part of their bodies well wrapped. They should wear a woolen shawl about their shoulders, have a woolen rug to draw over their knees and wind a band of flannel about their hips, as was done in earlier days. They must keep out of drafts and make sure their shoulders are well covered during sleep. When they feel pains coming on, they should resort to a hot-water bottle, whose gentle heat is both comforting and curative.

The best tisanes for rheumatism should be at once diuretic and pain-relieving. There is one I recommend to people with chronic arthritis. It is made with four slices of lemon, one pinch of lavender and one pinch of couch grass root boiled in a quart of water. This should be drunk at the rate of four cups a day, and not only during a bad spell but also when one is feeling better. When the pains are particularly acute, one may alternate this with another infusion consisting of one pinch of camomile, one pinch of lavender, two pinches of dried violets and two pinches of sage blossom—this for a quart of water. Again, this should be drunk at the rate of four cups a day. These are herbs that can counter the pain.

There are also methods for alleviating the pain by external treatments. I imagine that there are more salves, lotions, rubs and liniments for rheumatism than for any other illness. A number of these preparations are highly effective, as experience has proved.

My own experience convinces me that cabbage is of prime value against this group of infirmities. I will not repeat all I said in Chapter 3 on this subject, or recapitulate the various recipes given there. Let me only emphasize that cabbage excels all other vegetables in drawing out the pain of any inflammation, whether internal or external. It is also an easy vegetable to come by.

You can also try a pack of chopped cress or chopped chard, softened in boiling water. Similar results may be obtained from creeping ivy, peppermint, violet leaves or black briony (also known as Our Lady's Seal). You may prefer wet dressings prepared by dipping cloths in a decoction of these plants.

Other herbs are conveniently distilled into oil—these include camomile, marjoram and savory. Heat a pint of olive oil in a double boiler. Add 100 grams of any of the above herbs and continue heating for an hour. Strain. Frequent rubbings of the painful joint with this unguent will bring relief.

Sage and rosemary are also recommended as pain-killers. A bouquet of either in a very hot bath will ease the twinges.

There are also a number of old wives' prescriptions which, though lacking any scientific explanation, are reputed to keep rheumatism at bay. In Chapter 4 in the section on nettles I discussed some of these beliefs. If you want to immunize yourself against rheumatism, flog yourself with a bunch of nettles now and then. I admit this calls for a bit of courage.

You may also take up sleeping on a mattress stuffed with dried fern or dried elder leaves. This, too, is supposed to avert rheumatism. Old country people sometimes keep a particularly fine chestnut in their pocket, and will insist that this protects them against sciatica and gout.

If this seems far-fetched to you, I will attest that I knew a great surgeon who kept a length of hemp around his ankle to fend off rheumatism and that this talisman seemed to do its work.

There are some countries where people wear a copper bracelet on the theory that the magnetic effect of the metal serves to repel the various forms of rheumatism. One Japanese firm has mass-produced such bracelets for export throughout the globe. That no one so far has discovered the scientific or rational explanation for such phenomena does not in the least diminish their validity. Let us remember that for a long time the practice of acupuncture was considered pure superstition and witchery, yet Western medical experts who have watched it recently pronounce it a remarkable anesthetic technique in the most difficult operations.

I am acquainted with an Englishwoman who treats arthritis and rheumatism by bee stings. Similar experiments are going on in Germany and the Soviet Union. It is a carefully controlled procedure, both as to the number of stings and the parts of the body involved. When I was a five-year-old child I had an encounter with a swarm of bees and was stung all over. My father quickly rubbed me with an antivenom herb, which may have been either parsley or lavender, thyme or tomato leaves. I did not die of those stings and perhaps I owe my freedom from rheumatism to them. It is an interesting fact that the incidence of rheumatism is remarkably low among bee-keepers and honey producers. Short of keeping one's own hive, it might be a good thing to gently stroke a bee from time to time.

The Respiratory Tract

No illnesses are as common and as bothersome as the colds, flu and sore throats that plague us every year in cold weather. Despite the new vaccines that are just beginning to be used, these afflictions cost countless hours of lost working days and endless, if minor, discomfort.

Even if we cannot stamp out these troubles completely, we can at least keep them at a minimum by observing certain health rules. Once we are stricken, we can also do what is necessary to speedily get back on our feet.

A number of plants can be included in our diet and program of body care to build up our resistance against germs. I have already discussed the aromatic herbs used in the Vinegar of the Four Robbers—plants powerful enough to fend off the plague.

Present-day researchers have discovered antibiotic elements in no less than eight hundred forms of plant life. A goodly number of these are seaweeds and mushrooms, but similar properties are found in the modest mosses carpeting woods and uplands and in certain trees, particularly the pines. Among the edible plants, garlic is outstanding.

We can generally identify an antiseptic plant by its strong perfume. The list includes lavender, mint, thyme, rosemary, sage, eucalyptus, savory, citronella, clove, cinnamon, bergamot. Regular use of these herbs, both internally and externally, will keep germs away. Simply having them near is beneficial. Thus the Landes district of France, a region rich in pines, where the air is always fragrant with the scent of resin, is especially salubrious for people with weak lungs and children with delicate bronchi.

If microbes do invade your body, you must at once take steps to build up your resistance. As soon as you suspect you are coming down with a cold, try and work up a good sweat, for perspiration drives out toxins. Hot drinks are indicated. We all enjoy doctoring ourselves with grog, but alcohol is not always so well tolerated in illness. Certain tisanes will also produce a sweat: camomile, lavender, rosemary, thyme, the flower of borage and elderberry blossom. After drinking your tisane, you should heighten its effect by wrapping yourself in blankets or putting on heavier clothing.

Should you feel feverish, there are plants to combat that. First and foremost is garlic, but you would rather have that in a soup than in a tea, I would imagine. Then there is the ever dependable camomile, lemon, eucalyptus, centaury and wormwood, which is the flavoring agent of absinthe but is a useful medicinal herb in its own right.

It is sometimes advisable to go on a liquid diet consisting of vegetable soups, tisanes and fruit juices rich in vitamin C. Orange juice and hot lemonade are the classic recommendations.

Another trick to bring additional warmth to throat and chest is to apply a poultice to these areas. Old-fashioned country people would make up some linseed mash, potato starch or mustard paste for this purpose. Today the pharmacy offers more sophisticated mixtures. I recommend a pack of grated black radish or of chopped garlic, if the smell does not disturb you. Chopped oregano also makes a good revulsive.

By now you have a fairly good idea of the kind of cold you have. Only a simple head cold? You want to clear your head and your blocked nasal passages. A sneeze can bring comfort and there are herbs that help produce it. Sniff powdered marjoram and powdered sage. But the preferred way to clear these passages is to use an inhalator. The same effect can be achieved by breathing in the steam from a boiling infusion, with a towel draped over your head to concentrate the steam. The pharmacy supplies excellent inhalants based on eucalyptus gum. You can also make one yourself with an infusion of marjoram, thyme, rosemary and sage.

If the cold should settle at the throat and cause tonsillitis and coughing, gargles are very much in order. Our grandmothers used to prepare a honey of roses which is ideal for this purpose. You will find a recipe for it in Chapter 8. A strong decoction of blackberry leaves is also efficacious. You may use strawberry or raspberry leaves in the same way—that is, 50 grams of the leaves to a quart of water. Sweeten the liquid with honey. Another soothing gargle may be made from mallow leaves. Do not forget the four-flower tea (which is really a six-flower tea) mentioned in Chapter 4. Ground ivy, from which an extract is drawn for a commercial cough syrup, may also be used as an infusion. There is a plant aptly named lungwort that may be cooked in a soup along with cress and turnip leaves to supply nutrients especially useful during colds.

Should you lose your voice, I recommend something that may startle you: chew two or three plump cloves of garlic in the morning. An extreme thing to do, but after all it is hard to function without your voice. If this seems too much to ask, you have the alternative of drinking a tisane of hedge mustard, whose reputation for benefiting the voice is long and distinguished. There is a letter from Racine to Boileau in which he speaks of a choir singer at Notre Dame who was cured of a tragic loss of voice by drinking a tisane of hedge mustard. In bygone years people would concoct a syrup of hedge mustard and keep it on hand for emergencies. Here is the recipe: Boil 30 grams of hedge mustard leaves in a quart of water, reduce by two-thirds, add half a pound of sugar and flavor with liquorice.

As for me, when a cold strikes me (I am not entirely immune to them), I make a special tisane with plants my father used to favor for this purpose. It consists of a pinch of sage, a pinch of thyme and one of nettles. I drink two generous cups of this each day and sometimes that is all I need to feel tiptop again.

Allergies

Allergies are the more unnerving because their cause is hard to pin down. Perhaps these illnesses are on the increase these days. I call them illnesses because they can pretty well spoil life for those who have them. It is generally believed that the presence of chemicals in our food and the pollution of our environment have led to the incredible proliferation of allergies.

Their variety is infinite. Doctors who specialize in this field have at least a hundred vials in their cabinet for making tests: all manner of pollens, all manner of foods from eggs to strawberries, from wheat to chocolate, all sorts of feathers and hairs from domestic animals and household pets, ordinary household dust and rare dusts of this or that substance, fibers of wool, silk, cotton and synthetic textiles, detergents, dyes, shampoos, cosmetics, etc. It is a job for a detective to track down the guilty elements. The patient's symptoms offer hardly any clue. The usual signs are asthma, hay fever, eczema, rashes and other skin problems. To be sure, we know that hay fever is usually caused by pollens, rashes by some foodstuff, and eczema either by a cosmetic product or external contact. But these rules are not hard and fast and only represent the first step in the search.

Some people are predisposed to allergies. The susceptibility seems to a certain degree to be hereditary. Sometimes a family will have one parent who is asthmatic, while one of the children has hay fever and another is subject to rashes. Sometimes the original cause of the allergy lies far back in time and seems to have no connection with the patient's present tribulations.

One of my clients consulted me about her persistent hay fever. She had already been treated by a well-known allergist, who had put her through a series of tests in order to discover which pollen was responsible for her condition. It was plain that a pollen was involved, for her hay fever would unfailingly recur every year from the first of May to the end of June. Yet the patient manifested a normal reaction to all the test pollens tried on her.

The allergist, however, would not give up. Since the patient's hay fever could not be traced to any of the common grasses, he tried the more exotic plants. Suddenly he was brought up short by an unusually virulent reaction on the part of the patient. The test pollen came from a plant called ragweed, which is unknown on the continent of Europe but widely distributed throughout the United States. And in fact the young woman had spent some time in California, ten years earlier. But who would think of reviewing all one's trips, any more than of reporting what kind of fur coat one owns, or what cats one has stroked or the composition of one's pillows? After taking shots for three years with a special vaccine prepared by the Pasteur Institute, the young woman was still bothered by this violent allergy to a plant growing on some distant shore. I, too, could do little to help her until I managed to desensitize her organism by foot baths and hand baths. I drew on a wide range of plants: garlic for robustness; fresh celandine, that sometimes dangerous little flower which can work miracles; couch grass; sage; hawthorn; nerve-calming linden and others.

I treat asthma with a combination of common fruits and vegetables. Again I depend on garlic and, with it, lettuce (in a salad or braised), onions, cabbage, apples and grapes. During severe attacks I recommend a tisane of poppy to help the patient sleep. I recommend parsley as an expectorant, thyme for drying up the nasal phlegm, lavender, sage, celandine and ground ivy, which is particularly good for pulmonary ills of any sort.

I have devised a special drink, which has had excellent results, consisting of 5 grams of garlic, 5 grams of lemon, a pinch of mint blossom and a pinch of sage. This is steeped in a quart of boiling water and drunk at the rate of two cups a day. The taste may be odd but that is not important when asthma is in question. I have another curious-tasting drink I recommend for hay fever: 20 grams of garlic, 20 grams of onion and a pinch of violets.

To my mind, it seems entirely logical to turn to plants to

counterbalance the harm caused by other plants. The spring months can be trying to some of us, for nature fills the air with powerful essences which not everyone can bear. The solution is to find the plants that are well disposed toward you and avoid the ones that do you harm. The good plants will go to work at once to set your total organism to rights. But as my father used to say, it takes generations to acquire the lore to distinguish among the plants, with knowledge being handed down from father to son.

Nervous Complaints

As far back as my earliest memories go, the healing herbs have had a place in my life. My first lesson in herbs came when I was about three years old. My trouble was nerves and there were nights when I could not sleep. On such occasions my father would give me a special kind of bath. We had a big copper tub in the house which was used for canning. Father would fill it with warm water and throw in a generous handful of linden leaves. Then it would be set to warm to body temperature. Father would immerse me completely in this bath, except for my head, and keep me there for some time. I recall rather resenting this procedure. But Father would be right there and would say coaxingly: "Doesn't that feel good, my little one? It is a linden bath. Afterwards you will have no trouble sleeping."

I would actually start to doze off while still in the water. Mother would carry me to my bed sound asleep and I would have pleasant dreams about fairies who were really herbs and could cure all ills.

Nervous tension, which in past days was generally shortlived and due to special circumstances, is now unfortunately the regular condition for a good many people. It is the price we pay for modernity. Everyone is hurried and rushes about without knowing just why or where. In the slightest pause between activities people reach for the nearest stimulant: tea, coffee, cigarettes, and some, even drugs. At night, of course, they have trouble falling asleep and must resort to pills. They wake in the morning with a heavy head and need extra-strong coffee, or a pep pill, to be able to face the day. Then, naturally, their sleeping pills become even more necessary at night. They have embarked on a vicious circle that continues until the moment when their physique can no longer take the strain. Then they experience a depressive state, with the sense of total exhaustion and unrelieved blackness.

I have had a long procession of such people pass through my waiting room, some overwrought, some torpid. They have begged me to help them recover the natural rhythm of the days and nights, of work and repose.

My first instructions to them are that they must give up their dreadful habits and renounce both their sleeping pills and their stimulants, their tea, coffee, alcohol, tobacco and battery of pepper-uppers which, usually, they have no doctor's prescription for but take at random, deciding on the doses arbitrarily.

I next instruct them to revise their way of life, to settle on a simple healthful diet with regular meals, to get some exercise and to go to bed early, for the greatest profit is derived from sleep during the night hours and not from slumbering late in the morning.

Only after all these conditions have been fulfilled do I start my patients on a regime of calming herbs. My greatest standby is linden. Besides a linden bath of the sort I have described, there is linden tea, which taken in the evening will hardly fail to work its spell. There is also a tea of orange and hawthorn blossom that clears the head. It is especially valuable for women in their fifties troubled by hot flashes and migraine.

You can make an excellent mixed tea with a pinch of hawthorn blossom, a pinch of linden, a pinch of marjoram and 20 grams of lettuce leaves. Steep this in a quart of boiling water and drink four cups per day. You may remember that lettuce, included in your evening meal either as a salad or in cooked form, will help you get to sleep.

Give thought to the little poppy that grows so profusely in wheat fields and brightens the roadside with its scarlet. It is the modest cousin of the oriental poppy from which opium is made. One of my journalist friends has a Eurasian wife who knows a good deal about the herbal secrets of the East. From her I learned a simple method for inducing sleep: rub the back at night with a solution of poppy petals steeped in water. The active principle in the flower works at once on the nerves of the spinal cord and sleep is not long in coming.

I use the field poppy in various hand baths and foot baths, as well as in teas along with other calming herbs. Here is one such drink that has proved a boon to many insomniacs: one-half a pinch of poppy petals, 10 grams of lettuce leaves (this is the equivalent of two generous pinches of other herbs, but fresh lettuce is somewhat hard to measure by pinches), a pinch of hawthorn blossoms and a pinch of clover blossom. Steep in a quart of boiling water. You may need two cups of this at bedtime but the results are guaranteed.

Suppose you have had a good night's sleep behind you but you feel drowsy and lazy in the morning. There are ways to wake yourself up gently without recourse to tea or coffee, both of which impose a certain strain on the heart. Try a tea of sage or rosemary, of thyme or savory—or try alternating all four, using a pinch of each to the cup of boiling water. These aromatic herbs raise the energy level both physically and mentally.

You might substitute a cup of mint tea for the usual after-dinner coffee. It combats that tendency to drowsiness that comes after a hearty meal and aids in the process of digestion. But do not overdo the mint at night, unless you mean to make love. For mint directly feeds those inclinations.

Sexual Problems

In my youth people hardly spoke about "those matters." In our village women were modest and men inhibited. Nevertheless, from time to time I would catch a few words that would puzzle me. Once, for instance, a substantial citizen came to see my father and I overheard him saying: "My good Camille, I need your help. I can no longer pay honor to the ladies."

For a long time I wondered what sort of thing had to be done to pay honor to the ladies and how my father's herbs could help a man learn good manners. But after twenty-five years of experience as a healer, I must sorrowfully admit that men—and women, too—have a great deal to learn in this domain and that there seem to be more and more problems complicating the relationship between the sexes.

I have been told tales that strained the imagination and stories to make one weep. I have offered my counsel to men suffering from impotence and to women suffering from frigidity, to homosexuals, to girls still in their teens but already hardbitten with sexual experience, to sadists and people with every sort of quirk and perversion. Some of these cases I was able to help not only by my treatments but also by our talks together. For many people with this sort of problem cannot discuss it with their families or with their doctor. I was able to win their confidence, and this was the first step toward a cure.

The most common complaint of men was impotence, and with this impairment of their virility, their entire self-respect would crumble. But impotence, unless arising from a serious organic condition, is often only temporary and can be traced either to health deficiencies or painful psychological factors. In both these contingencies there is much that can be done to bring improvement.

Sometimes there is no actual impotence, only an absence of desire. This may occur in men who have practiced masturbation for long periods of time and feel only disgust for the procedures of love.

There is a third category of men who suffer from insufficient sexual control and can sustain an erection for only the briefest time. Knowing beforehand that they can bring only disappointment to their partner, they feel frustration and resentment.

In all three cases we want to remake the man from a poor lover into a great one. But a great lover is not created in a single day.

The substantial citizen who came to see my father because he could no longer pay honor to the ladies would first have had to get rid of his paunch. For age is not always responsible for loss of erotic capacity. There are young men whose prowess in this realm is small and older men who are champions in bed.

My first advice is take up some sort of sport in order to strengthen the muscles and improve the circulation. In addition, it might be well to follow the example of athletes, keeping away from alcohol, tobacco and coffee. Voltaire called coffee the beverage of eunuchs. And a Persian king, who wanted to subdue too spirited a stallion, instructed the stable attendants: "Have the horse drink coffee." Slander, to be sure, will have it that the king was speaking out of personal experience. As for diet, make sure you have good meat, preferably beef, as well as fish and shellfish. Eat plenty of fruits and green vegetables, especially celery and fennel, but do not eat too heavily.

Good roosters are thin, the country people say. I have found virility is highest among men who do physical labor, among country dwellers and among the poor. Blacks, who by and large meet these conditions, are well known to be stalwart lovers. By contrast intellectuals, city people and men who have grown portly on prosperity are often prone to difficulties in this area of life.

The search for a potion which would endow the user with sexual energy seems to be as old as civilization. We have records of some very bizarre recipes that enjoyed great favor at one or another period in history, only to drop totally out of sight thereafter. Nevertheless, there was often something to these preparations.

Nostradamus, the celebrated sixteenth-century astrologer, recommended a recipe that called for mandrake root, among other things, as well as the blood of male sparrows, the tentacles of squid, ambergris, cinnamon, musk, clove, honey and Cretan wine. While some of the ingredients seem to have only exotic value, others, like cinnamon and cloves, do have aphrodisiac qualities. As for ambergris, it occurs frequently in such aphrodisiacs, in a more recent era in the famous chocolate concocted by Brillat-Savarin to heighten the potency of bons-vivants.

Some of these potions are based on the theory of resemblance. Thus eating shellfish would promote virility because of the resemblance of the mollusk to the female genitals. Nowadays we still believe that shellfish and lobster promote sexual activity, but chiefly because these foods are rich in certain proteins.

Another ingredient in the past would be the testicles of various animals. There was also a preference for rare and precious spices: pimento, pepper, paprika, nutmeg, cinnamon, cloves. In fact, these spices do sharpen the senses, provided they are not used too often.

Last but not least came the truffle, to which miracles were ascribed. But for it, King Henri IV of France might not have been born, for history recounts that his good mother had eaten *pâté de foie gras* with truffles the day he was conceived. As for Napoleon, though no one can question his sexual prowess, he was not especially fertile. His cook Curnonsky, who has recounted some revealing little anecdotes about the emperor, has something to say on this matter:

> Before the birth of the King of Rome, Napoleon was much concerned at having no heir. Word came to him of one of his officers who spawned bastards right and left. He had the man sent for and asked him the secret of his fecundity. "Sire," the fellow replied, "I dine beforehand on turkey stuffed with truffles and have a bottle of dry champagne." Napoleon followed this program—and it was not long before the young queen was in the family way.

Curnonsky has another comment to make on the subject of truffles. "Properly speaking," he writes, "there are no aphrodisiacs capable of endowing those blind to love with sight. But for those with poor eyesight in this matter, there are substances which act as magnifying lenses."

This corresponds to my view of the question. I do not promise miracles but I can offer the possibility of amelioration. And since a truffle cure is somewhat beyond the means of most of us, let me urge the merits of a democratic garlic cure, for garlic is a great restorative of vigor.

I had occasion to prescribe garlic to an actor who was in love with a young actress but seemed unable to give a proper accounting of himself. After a while he came to see me again. "I have a new problem, Mességué," he said. "We can't seem to stop. Don't you have something to calm me down?"

Women, too, come to me with their sexual problems. For the most part these are directly connected with the inadequacies of their husbands or lovers. Hence it is advisable to treat both members of a couple. Many women are frigid simply because the man in their life has never known how to make them vibrate. As Balzac put it: "When it comes to love, woman is a lyre and yields her music to him who knows how to play her strings."

To a couple with sexual problems I therefore say: "Have a little wedding feast together from time to time, and season your dishes with truffles or garlic, as you think best. Help each other prepare the simple herb potions whose recipes I'll give you and the herbal preparations with which you will rub each other's body as a prelude to your sweet caresses. For to share a concern, a hope, and an effort is in itself to share love. Trust in the outcome and you will not be disappointed."

Go out to the country together and ramble in the fields, hand in hand, looking for what my father used to call the herbs of happiness. Look for the lacy Queen Anne's lace, the pungent savory, the various mints that love to grow by brooks, fenugreek, the golden flower of the celandine and the musky rocket. Later have yourselves a few cups of the following tisane whose taste will make you laugh: 5 grams of garlic and 5 of onion, a pinch of savory and a pinch of mint—this to a quart of water. Or, somewhat less odd-tasting, this other tisane: a pinch of the root of Queen Anne's lace, a pinch of savory, a half-pinch of nettles and a half-pinch of corn silk.

Here is a simple preparation for your massages: two pinches of celandine plus one of fenugreek to be steeped in a quart of cold water. Let it sit for twenty-four hours, then rub the small of the back with a cotton wad dipped in this solution.

For women I recommend a daily douche with the following solution: a pinch of sage, four pinches of mallow and two pinches of dried violet blossoms. The effect is highly refreshing, and any young woman in love, or hoping to be, should make this part of her beauty routine.

To be sure, the sexual mechanism of women is extremely complicated and they suffer from a host of troubles that play havoc with their emotional life. But in this matter, too, herbs can come to their aid. There are herbs that can speed a tardy menstruation: parsley, which can be added to vegetable juice and marigold flowers, which makes a pleasant tisane. Those herbs that are useful against hemorrhaging will also control a too copious flow: shepherd's purse, geranium and horsetail.

Nowadays we have reason to believe that certain herbs contain substances closely related to the female hormones. The richest in these is sage, which can serve as a tonic to the uterus. Hops is another plant that has a conspicuous effect on sexual functioning. In hop-growing regions the women who pick the hops absorb some element by osmosis and find their menstrual cycles interrupted during the harvest season. In Holland the women who sort and pack tulip bulbs experience a similar reaction.

Such plants have been branded abortifaciants, but this is overstating the case. The most they do is bring on or slow down the period. In fact, I would say that they favor fertility insofar as they can regulate this sometimes capricious rhythm.

For any vaginal inflammation I recommend a series of douches with infusions of soothing decongestive mallow.

Finally, if men or women are troubled like my friend the actor with too violent and too wearing desires, they may turn for help to the calming herbs I mentioned in my chapter on insomnia. There is also that most antiaphrodisiac of plants, the water lily. Since the Middle Ages it has been known as the plant of chastity, and all sorts of syrups, potions and sweetmeats were made of it. These were much favored by monks and pious nuns for banishing unclean dreams. But nowadays there is little demand for water-lily syrup.

The Heart and the Circulatory System

There was one fine gentleman who used to visit my father once a year during the harvest season. He came from quite a distance, from a little village in the Pyrenees of which he was the mayor. But my father used to address him as *Monsieur le Président* to show his respect. I was also in enormous awe of him, first because he was such a big man and so ruddy, but also because he arrived by car, a luxury in those days, and came with Dr. Echernier, who was in his own right a person of great importance and my father's most illustrious acquaintance. Imagine—a doctor!

In view of the high status of these visitors my father used to tell my mother to prepare holiday fare—*coq au vin*, partridges and capons, *foie gras* and a number of desserts. I can still see our guest licking his lips over the *foie gras*, and sweating profusely as he gorged himself on all these good things. My father, too, would watch him stuff himself and when they came to the dessert would tell him respectfully but firmly: "Well, *Monsieur le Président*, this is the last good meal you are going to have. Tomorrow you start on your diet."

For this glutton suffered from hypertension, which was the reason he came to consult my father. This last heavy meal had some of the ritual meaning of the last cigarette for a condemned criminal. From the next day on, this man was going to be restricted to one slice of veal with three cloves of garlic and three onions. Besides this, he would be allowed only some boiled vegetables, salads and fruits. He might also drink a few tisanes that my father would prescribe.

Dr. Echernier was in charge of the patient and would keep my father abreast of his progress. After a month the news would be that he was getting better. His weight would be down and his blood pressure approaching normal. But as the months went on, he would begin to break the rules. And by the time the harvest season had rolled around again, there he was, potbellied and short of breath, come to consult my father. My father gave him the usual scolding, my mother prepared the usual last feast, and so on.

So it goes. If people did not overeat, heart disease would not be the scourge it is. But as things stand, it is the number one cause of death in prosperous countries. Abundance is a blessing, but we pay dearly for it.

After a certain age hypertension is a fairly common complaint. Its symptoms are various: dizziness, buzzing in the ear, palpitations. In the course of time the condition tires the heart. The first imperative is to change one's eating habits in favor of a diet low in red meat, starches and fats. The patient should forgo both alcohol and coffee, while salt and spices should be severely restricted or even entirely eliminated.

While I am a strong believer in the value of sports, I have reservations where people with heart problems are concerned, For them the best thing is walking at a moderate and steady pace; violent sports that cause shortness of breath should be avoided. Similarly, they should eschew hot baths in favor of warm baths or even sponge baths.

This does not mean that I would condemn heart patients to a lifetime of near-starvation. The veal-onion-garlic routine is only meant as a shock treatment, to be followed for a limited time. Nevertheless, I would insist that garlic be given a prominent place in their future eating patterns. That garlic counteracts the effects of cholesterol has been recognized by medicine. Those who object to the robust taste of this condiment can buy a garlic extract at the pharmacy. Those, however, who enjoy its unique flavor might try the following recipe: Put a pound of garlic through the juicer. Mix the juice with an equal quantity of alcohol. Take two or three spoonfuls of this daily. If you follow such a garlic cure for one week every month, you will keep hypertension at bay.

There are many plants that benefit the heart, calming and regulating a disordered heartbeat. First and foremost of these is the hawthorn, which corrects palpitations. Two or three pinches of dried hawthorn blossom to a quart of water makes a useful infusion. The leaves of the olive tree (twenty leaves boiled in a cup of water) are also effective. Lily of the valley (one pinch of the flowers to a cup of water) has a regulatory effect on the heart, as does mint. Finally, there is the foxglove, from which digitalis is extracted. But this is a more powerful medicine and should not be taken except under medical supervision.

I recommend the following tisane for hypertension: two pinches of hawthorn blossom, one pinch of lavender blossom and 5 grams of garlic—this to a quart of water. Drink two cups of this per day.

Another method for relieving palpitations is to apply compresses to the heart, the cloth dipped in a strong infusion of the following plants: a handful of hawthorn blossom, a handful of celandine (the entire plant, as fresh as possible), a handful of buttercup (stems and leaves, and a handful of heather. Let the mixture steep a while. It may be kept and used for several days, being warmed anew each time.

Another unfortunate concomitant of age is arteriosclerosis, or hardening of the arteries. A strict diet should be followed. I also recommend the following drink, which is almost a soup: 5 grams of garlic, 5 grams of onion and a pinch of dandelion— this to a quart of water. Drink four cups of this per day.

Circulatory troubles may be present without any heart disorder. These often afflict women during pregnancy or during the menopause. For them I recommend a tisane that stimulates the circulation: a pinch of parsley, a pinch of sage, a pinch of marigold flowers and a half-pinch of dock root—this to a quart of water. Drink two cups a day.

Bad circulation is also responsible for such problems as hemorrhoids, varicose veins, varicose ulcers, etc. These minor ailments may be treated simultaneously by internal and external means.

Horse chestnut figures prominently in the composition of certain suppositories that soothe varicose veins and hemorrhoids. Why not, then, make direct use of this common nut, which every child knows and enjoys collecting. Peel away its tough skin and set it to boil, using 10 grams of the nut to the quart of water. The beverage does not taste very good, but becomes tolerable with the addition of a little sugar. A drink with similar properties may be made from the bark of the chestnut tree, using 30 grams of bark to a quart of water.

Even bitterer is a brew made of pine bark but its virtues as a remedy for varicose veins and hemorrhoids are acknowledged. It is prepared in the same fashion as the chestnut bark preparation.

An effective compound may be made by mixing these two plants with that interesting plant, horsetail. Again, the recipe calls for ten minutes of boiling, in view of the toughness of the material. The proportions are 2 grams of peeled horse chestnut, 2 grams of pine bark and two pinches of horsetail (the entire plant)—this to a quart of water. Drink two cups per day.

All these solutions may be used in more highly concentrated doses as external medicaments, either for bathing the hemorrhoidal tissues or for applying as warm wet dressings on the varicose veins. Several other plants are useful for reducing varicosity. These are knapweed, sage and walnut bark. Strong decoctions of these plants—50 grams of the plant material to a quart of water—may be used to wash open wounds and speed their healing.

In the past richness of blood used to be considered an index of health. Nowadays such richness is often the cause of our ills. Yet the opposite condition, thin blood, is still among us in the form of anemias of various sorts. The usual sufferers are young children, convalescents and the elderly.

How can we restore color to the cheeks of a pale, anemic

person? Through garlic, I say, always through garlic. I am not ashamed of repeating myself on this subject, for I cannot recommend garlic strongly enough. Both children and old people should be given it, as they should be given those other vitalizing vegetables like cabbage, spinach and celery. Their languid appetites may be stimulated by black radish. Among the fruits, the best of all is apricot, which contains more vitamins than cod-liver oil (which in my own youth was heartily detested by children). A valuable herb for its tonic and appetite-building properties is gentian. A delicious wine may be made from it—the recipe is given in Chapter 8. There is also water trefoil, which prevents rickets in children and is rich in assorted vitamins. You may want to take it as a tisane—one pinch to a cup of water.

In this day and age we should all know our blood type, just as naturally as we know our name, age and address. We should have this notation on our person at all times, in our wallet or memo book. In case of accident and the necessity of a blood transfusion such information saves a great deal of time.

Let me urge the desirability of a yearly health checkup for everyone over forty. The checkup should include a blood analysis through which imbalances may be discovered. Problems such as excessive cholesterol, albumen or urea in the blood, or disturbances in the blood-sugar level (diabetes) will come to light through such a test. Treated early, these conditions may be corrected by means of diet, but if they are neglected, they quickly reach an advanced stage and lead to dangerous consequences.

Perhaps our foremost aim in caring for our health should be to maintain the fluidity and youthfulness of the blood. The functioning of all the organs ultimately depends on the quality of the blood. And through the ages has not the heart been taken as the symbol of life itself?

6. Beauty: A Promise of Happiness

The fine town ladies used to come to see my father in secret. I would be watching from behind the curtain as they stepped down from their carriages, their feet encased in tight high-heeled shoes, their figures confined by corsets and their faces hidden by a wisp of veiling. They would pretend to be out for a drive in the country and simply dropping in on Camille Mességué for a social chat. Father was almost always available. Except for market day, when there might be a goodly number of people in town who would want to consult him, his waiting room was not crowded. To be accurate, Father had no proper waiting room but saw his patients wherever was most convenient, either indoors or out.

The ladies, however, would be ushered indoors, for Father understood their preference for discretion. I remember one of them who struck me as especially elegant. Her face was perfectly immobile, so that she seemed to be following the principle of Baudelaire's Hymn to Beauty:

> I hate any movement that ruffles my features.
> I never weep and I never laugh.

But this type of beauty seems to have had its day. Nowadays what we most appreciate is beauty in motion.

Sometimes an elderly gentleman would drop by to see my father. I would notice how well groomed he looked, not at all like the country people, and I would hear Father discussing flowers and perfumes with him. There was also a military officer who was exceedingly careful of his appearance. Father always addressed him as Colonel. (Perhaps he was only a captain, but Father tended to promote people a couple of ranks.)

What these various people had in common was that they were not sick. Rather, they were concerned about their physical ap-

154

pearance. They wished either to become beautiful or to retain their beauty. As for me, I soon came to recognize another distinction in Father's practice. When Father went out to the fields with his old black razor, the kind used by old-fashioned barbers, he intended to cut nettles, ivy or couch grass to make up some remedy for his sick patients. But when he took his white razor, the one with the mother-of-pearl handle, he was going to do something for his other clientele.

It was the white razor Father used to cut roses whose petals went into beauty preparations. Father favored yellow roses for this purpose. I would hurry to put on my *sabots* and go with him. The roses could not be picked after a rain, or when the dew was on them or when the sun was high. The best time was about ten o'clock in the morning. Father's face would have a special joyous look when he was cutting roses.

I would help him, sorting the petals, removing any that were in the least spoiled or discolored. "We'll need three hundred petals," he would tell me, "for the blue bottle there." I would start counting patiently, but Father would soon intervene. He could judge quantities by eye. The petals would be set to steep in rain water. Father would wipe the razor dry, close it and put it carefully away in its customary drawer. And in a few days one of the ladies would appear, or else one of Father's gentlemen clients, and would be given the rosewater along with some discreet instructions on how to use it.

His whole life long Father had pursued the secrets of beauty and youth. Like Dr. Faust, he engaged in experiments and was continually improving his methods. While he was perfectly willing to say what went into his remedies, he would become rather secretive in regard to the beauty preparations. One reason I became interested in this field is that I was impressed very early by the aura of mystery surrounding the subject. In fact, the science of beauty is still only in its early stages.

Over the years Father had developed certain formulas which he kept strictly to himself. When I was old enough to understand, he told me: "My dear son, I am not a rich man but I have something to leave you which will make your fortune, if you know how to use it. It will also enable you to do a great deal of good. Women, especially, will bless you, for you will be able to make them beautiful. You will leave this formula to your children and they will bequeath it to theirs."

Every so often Father would wink at me and say, to whoever was around: "The boy knows a secret which will make him a bigwig—a bigwig, I tell you!"

While I was at work on this book a letter came to me from Irma D., who had been a good friend of our family. She is now a charming old lady living in Monfaucon, a village outside of Rabastens. This is what she wrote:

> My dear Maurice,
>
> Who is this person who addresses you in such a familiar tone? An old granny of seventy-one who knew you from the time you were four. Who knew and loved your whole family. Back then, we used to pack our togs and go and visit "with the Mességués." We generally would make the trip at harvest time and stay in Gavarret for about a month. How we all enjoyed it there! It was the best kind of holiday.
>
> I can see you all as you were then. I often remember something your father used to say. "Irma," he would tell me solemnly, "mark my words: Maurice will be a bigwig someday." He was perfectly right. How happy he would be to know of your career. He was such a dear person.

One other person besides me knew Father's secret. This was my mother. All through the years she religiously followed his recipes. After his death she would pay tribute to his memory by keeping up the rituals he had taught her. Though she is now in her seventies and has had all sorts of sorrows—widowhood and the hardships it brought, not to speak of the worries connected with my many lawsuits—she still looks amazingly youthful, with a lovely complexion, smooth skin and not a trace of wrinkles.

I felt I was carrying out the terms of Father's testament when I set up my Laboratory of Wild Herbs some fifteen years ago. Now I think I can reveal the secret my father left me without fear of its being stolen by my competitors. It is a beauty mask based on mallows, brambles and a homeopathic dose of celandine. I called it Essence of Youth 70—not because that was the year when I put it on the market but because my mother was seventy years old. I dedicated the beauty mask to her. My father would have wanted it that way.

In addition to balms, creams and lotions, Father had a great feeling for perfumes and would make some up for his clients. There would always be crocks of rainwater about the house in which flowers would be steeping. Father would blend special scents, supposedly with aphrodisiac properties, which he would dispense to his elderly gentlemen. His lady clients would also keep him informed of the effects of the perfumes he had created for them. Father would look very gratified.

Father himself always smelled of violets. All my memories of him are associated with this fragrance. I do not know if Father actually used a violet perfume or whether the smell was not somehow an emanation of him, the symbol of his predominant virtue, modesty. At any rate, it could not have been that "odor of sanctity" whose existence I learned of later and which seems to be a specific attribute of sainthood. Thus a gardener who was called to the deathbed of St. Theresa of Avila attested to the perfume given off by the great Carmelite: violet, jasmine and iris. In our own century Pope Pius IX was also reputed to give off a flower-like smell—the scent of carnation. These are, it would seem, conspicuous examples of a more general phenomenon scientists have had to take account of: that mystics, during a period of religious exaltation, produce certain chemical substances, each according to his physical nature, which are closely related to the perfumes produced by flowers. The odor of sanctity would appear to be an intensified form of this. I do not claim that Father's aroma of violets, or Mother's aroma of lavender or my own desire to surround myself with the scent of roses has anything to do with sainthood, but it is a fact that every individual has his particular perfume, which may either be innate or be absorbed from the plant in question. There are plants that leave their mark on us for some time after we have come into contact with them—one such example (a not very poetic one) is garlic. And cannot gourmets recognize the special taste of a rabbit that has fed on thyme or a honey made by bees that have browsed on rosemary?

In our family even the horse, Colibri, had his perfume. Colibri was a hard-working beast, particularly in the hay-making season. But he was snow-white and always as beautifully groomed as if he were being entered in a horse show. Father made up a special lotion for our horse, and when he went out to gather the materials for it, he would take the razor with the mother-of-pearl handle.

The local people were considerably impressed by Colibri's appearance and would come around to ask Father how he kept the horse looking so good. For selling purposes it always helped to have your animals sleek and shiny, for that was a sign of good health. So Father dispensed his beauty secrets for horses. The key plants were mistletoe and couch grass: one-fifth of the first and four-fifths of the second, to be mixed in their feed, and the same plants in maceration to be used as a rubdown.

Nowadays, when I am more and more occupied with this other aspect of my work, I realize how strong is the human desire for beauty. Women of every age will come immense distances, not because they are in ill health, but because they hope for some transformation from me. The impulse is apparently worldwide. Some years ago, when I was to appear on the Canadian radio, I found a number of Eskimo women waiting outside the broadcast studio, along with a missionary father. The latter had recently returned from France and had told his flock about Maurice Mességué. Apparently his female parishioners had been so struck by what they heard that they wanted to seek me out and ask me how they could achieve a peaches-and-cream complexion. But my most persistent clients are the Japanese, who are most concerned with perfumes that will bind their men to them.

I believe that in our times, when medicine has made such great strides and the knowledge of dietetics is so widely circulated, the great dream of women, and as a matter of fact of men, too, is to attain beauty and preserve the look of youth.

It was Stendhal who wrote: "Beauty is a promise of happiness." And is not the pursuit of happiness our great quest these days? What a procession of women have passed through my consulting room, distressed over this or that blemish, the beginning of wrinkles, some patches of cellulite, which they felt threatened to lose them their husbands. I am all for happy households: if all that is wanted is a cream to save these marriages, I am glad to supply it.

Meanwhile I keep on experimenting. I am only an artisan of beauty, as I am an artisan of health.

I am most concerned about two qualities in my creams and

preparations: that they be fresh and that they be made of pure materials only. Creams made with herbs that have been exposed to chemicals (insecticides, etc.) will block the pores of the skin rather than open them. Sooner than risk this, it is better to do without such beauty treatments. As for the freshness of a cream, this has considerable bearing on its usefulness. Stale preparations are almost no good at all. The best beauty products are those you can make yourself from the familiar plants in your garden, and apply at once. In the following sections you will find simple and efficacious recipes of this sort.

In the United States, where the pursuit of beauty and youth is more ardent, perhaps, than anywhere on earth, there is a movement afoot to return to natural patterns. Not only has gardening become the rage, with countless amateur vegetable-growers practicing the principles of organic farming, but there is also a strong bias in favor of natural cosmetics. The new purists want their lipsticks made without any chemical dyes, but taking their color from carrots, beets and currants. They want their creams and beauty masks made from such healthful substances as cucumbers, potatoes or strawberries, and their toothpaste made from eggplant. To be sure, this fad may well be justified in a country which has for too long lived in terms of artificialities and committed so many sins against nature. I would not ask for quite such sweeping measures but rather a strict control over the quality and freshness of the beauty products on the market. But if our pretty girls should one day decide they want to throw away their tubes of lipstick and color their lips with currant jelly, I would be the first to approve. I am sure they would look as lovely as ever.

Cellulite

Those times are gone when women laced themselves into corsets and disguised their shape with layers of petticoats. Nowadays all women, the young and the not-so-young, are through with such uncomfortable artifices. They want to wear a minimum of clothing, which will be both functional and flattering. But their dearest dream is to show themselves in a bikini on a beach.

Of course, a beautiful body in a bikini is an adorable sight and I would be the last to wish for more concealing beach wear. Nevertheless, the bikini is merciless toward any defect. For it unsparingly reveals those unfortunate bulges and paddings of fat that seem to settle by preference on the thighs, the hips, at the knees, around the ankles or the upper arms, even when there is nothing wrong with the rest of the silhouette.

How often young women have come to my office who seem confused, embarrassed about undressing and saddled with a permanent complex because of their cellulite. While men are prone to suffer from a paunch or from general fat that clothes their entire trunk like some sort of lifejacket, with women cellulite is far more common than plain obesity. These lumps and swellings are not caused by fat but by the retention of fluid.

It is hard to determine the causes of cellulite. With some, the root lies in an emotional shock, a death, an unhappy love affair, some obstruction in their professional life or simply long-standing nervous fatigue. In all these conditions toxins are created within the body which interfere with its proper functioning. With other people, there are physical causes for the condition: lack of exercise, insufficient fresh air and a faulty diet. The problem is not necessarily eating to excess but eating too many artificial and chemical products which the body refuses to assimilate.

In all these situations it is necessary to restore the body's equilibrium by good sleep, moderate exercise and general relaxation. Vacations can be a fine time to break the undesirable habits and carry out a cure that will detoxify the body. In addition, a diet should be followed. First and foremost the body must be cleansed of poisons. Any of the natural diuretics mentioned in previous chapters are suitable for this. This is the moment to make a cure with onions, celery, cucumber, cabbage, leeks, fennel, parsley or strawberries. You can drink tisanes of cherry stems or apple peelings, of borage or of meadowsweet. I highly recommend an infusion made of a pinch of dandelion, a pinch of couch grass, a pinch of corn silk—all this in a quart of water and drunk at the rate of four cups a day.

Besides the plants with strong diuretic properties, all the green vegetables and fresh fruits will be of help, provided they are free of chemicals. Hence it is important to avoid preserved forms of these foods and instead eat them in the fresh state.

It is also wise to eat high-protein meats, as lean as possible. Have them grilled and use herbs for seasoning. Veal and pork are less nutritious and are apt to be impregnated with artificial hormones and antibiotics. Poultry is good if the birds have been raised on pure grain. The same rule applies to eggs.

You will want to cut back on rich fare, fats, sugars and starches. Avoid fried foods, though you may have a bit of olive oil on your salad and a little cheese for a dessert. You may not have white sugar, either in jams or in baked stuffs. Instead use honey and fresh fruit which requires no sugaring, such as apples or grapefruit. Give up white bread, pies or cakes. A few slices of whole bread, however, are permitted. Use lemon instead of vinegar and herbs instead of salt and spices. Drink chicory or herbal teas instead of coffee, and mineral water instead of wine.

Along with these measures for internal detoxification, there are external treatments that will break down the globules of cellulite and smooth away unsightly puckerings. Massage is excellent. There are now many electrical devices for massage on the market, but I greatly prefer old-fashioned manual methods, which do no violence to the tissues. In this matter, as in so many others, I believe in human contact. For simplicity, warmth and sensitivity there is no machine that can equal the human hand.

I have experimented with a good many lotions against cellulite. Among the commercial products the majority are made with seaweed, but I prefer to use plants that grow on my own lands, and seaweed does not fit into that category. I have found that ivy is the most effective, and I have used it a thousand times and in any number of ways. I have made an anticellulite cream of it, but I also use it in wet dressings and compresses applied to the bulges. Ground ivy, crushed and rubbed into the skin or applied as a poultice for several hours, dissolves the globules of cellulite. You can also make a solution by steeping generous handfuls of ivy, either the climbing variety or ground ivy, in cold water for twenty-four hours. Use this as a wash and repeatedly bathe the patches of cellulite with it.

Finally, I make up hand and foot baths of my favorite anticellulite plants: celandine, couch grass, horsetail, buttercup and, of course, ivy. I place great value on such treatments by osmosis. If formulas of this sort seem to be missing here, it is because I have dealt with them in my previous book, *Of Men and Plants*, and do not want to repeat myself. Moreover, I usually make up these compounds for each individual patient and include certain plants in homeopathic doses. In this book my policy has been to give only prescriptions people can make up themselves, with easily obtainable materials and without any risks attached. My aim is not to flaunt my esoteric methods but on the contrary to give people simple directions for looking after their own health and happiness. To take care of oneself is part of being a responsible individual. It is a failure of responsibility to expect the doctor or the plant-healer to repeatedly correct the harm one has done one's body by neglect or misuse.

In his *Les Hommes en Blanc* ("Men in White") André Soubiran has made an observation I can second: "Do not imagine that stupid notions about medicine are a specialty of country bumpkins. If you want to hear a cultivated person speak absolute nonsense, ask him something about medicine."

If cultivated people along with country bumpkins were willing to stick to simple things, perhaps they would make fewer mistakes. To know a few herbs and to use them intelligently is already to be far ahead. Thus if women relied on roses for their faces, carrots for their stomachs and ivy for their figures, they would be well along on the road to beauty.

The Skin

A lithe and graceful body is now yours, thanks to a program of exercise and sensible eating. But what if your happiness is clouded by another kind of affliction, namely some skin eruption?

A skin condition can be a serious matter calling for the attention of a doctor. Furunculosis, psoriasis and eczema should all be treated by a dermatologist. Nevertheless, they can be considerably relieved by certain reforms in your diet.

In case of furunculosis your doctor will at once forbid you highly seasoned food, spices, sauces and any form of alcohol. But

I would advise you to also weigh your meals heavily in favor of those depurative vegetables that clean the blood. These are chicory, nettles, leeks and onions. Among the fruits, grapes lead the list.

You can speed the healing of the boils by applying poultices of cooked lettuce leaves or chopped cabbage, either raw or boiled, or lily bulbs cooked in milk. All the vegetables are known to be effective in this way.

You may also apply compresses dipped in solutions of thyme or sage or mallow. Or you might make up a solution of all three herbs, thus combining their virtues.

Eczema and herpes are sometimes of nervous origin. On the other hand, they may represent an allergy to a specific substance (some dye, cosmetic, synthetic fiber, etc.). Skin problems of this sort are greatly on the increase nowadays and their causes ever more difficult to trace. Let me repeat that insofar as you can avoid contact with chemicals whether in your food, your body care products or your clothing, you will be lessening the risk of troublesome skin reactions.

The patient with eczema is apt to report that there is asthma in his family or rheumatism or obesity—or all three. Conjunctions of this sort indicate a single underlying cause. What we have here is a chronic intoxication of nervous origin. The first requirement is to relax the nerves by exercise and sport, and detoxify the body by a purifying diet. However, when I advise such patients to go on a vacation, I stipulate that they should not go to the seashore. Water is bad for eczema and spreads the rash. Even baths and showers must be avoided. If the eczema is localized on the hands, I recommend that the patient wear rubber gloves when he is doing any dirty job so that he need not have to wash his hands afterward.

The diet should lean heavily on garlic, carrots, lettuce, onion and dandelion. Among the fruits, grapes are especially good. A cure of lemon juice (drunk several times iin the course of the day) is also highly beneficial. Of the depurative teas, the best is chicory. Include both leaves and roots, one pinch per cup. One may also make a tea from the root of the wild pansy, one pinch per cup, which is a useful medicament for skin troubles in general. I prescribe it for babies with cradle cap.

Burdock is another plant with curative properties against eczema. Prepare a lotion by boiling two pinches of the plant, either its leaves or root, for half an hour in a quart of water. Then wash the afflicted areas with this solution. Blackberry blossoms may be used similarly.

A traditional country remedy for eczema was to apply a paste made by boiling garlic, then mixing it with equal parts of honey. This would be smeared on and covered with a gauze bandage.

Psoriasis is a skin ailment that occurs chiefly on the elbows, knees and hands. Tiny pimples appear, each no larger than the head of a pin, but producing nasty itching. Sometimes the condition is caused by contact with rough fabrics, while in other cases the cause is considered to be certain detergents with a petroleum base. Of course, your best approach is to discover the real cause and eliminate it. Your doctor will be of help with this. But meanwhile it is important to adopt a sane light diet to detoxify the body. The vegetables recommended for liver disorders are highly suitable: artichoke, carrots, lettuce, leeks and beets.

Teas of borage, chervil or sage (one pinch per cup) are efficacious. The same infusions may also be used in wet dressings applied to the affected areas. I have had good results with a tea made with one pinch of camomile, one of sage and one of dandelion (the entire plant)—this to a quart of water and drunk at the rate of four cups per day.

It is particularly unfortunate when someone contracts a skin disease in the country when he has gone there for health purposes. Such rashes are usually short-lived and come about from gathering certain flowers like primroses and cowslips, to which some people are allergic. If you are sensitive in this respect, you had better forego the pleasure of picking flowers.

A program of body care will often prevent skin disease. I have already discussed the disinfectant properties of the aromatic herbs like thyme, rosemary and sage. Some sprigs of these, thrown into the bath, or made into infusions, cleanse and protect the skin. You can also blend yourself a gentle lotion out of one pinch of hawthorn blossom, two pinches of cornflowers, two pinches of camomile, two of lavender, two of mallow root and a fistful of rose petals. Steep these in two quarts of boiled water.

The famous beauties of history took great pains with their

toilette and especially with their skin. Some of their secrets have come down to us: Cleopatra would add ass's milk to her bath water, and others would use honey and almond oil. In our grandmothers' day a popular bath accessory was the bran bag, while various floral and herbal vinegars were favored for after-bath lotions to wash away any trace of lime left by the water and to stimulate circulation. The best-known of these was rose vinegar (100 grams of red rose petals steeped in a quart of white vinegar for fifteen days). However, you can make up similar lotions with lavender, with orange blossom, with citronella and with mint.

Almond oil is a time-honored balm for dry skins, and is especially good for diaper rash in babies. Familiar olive oil is also excellent for this purpose and makes, moreover, a first-rate suntan oil. You can prepare your own bronzing lotion by mixing one cup of purest olive oil with ten drops of iodine and the juice of a lemon. Shake the bottle well before applying to the skin. Olive oil is rich in vitamins and nourishes the epidermis. However, it attracts the sun's rays and would tend to produce sunburn were it not for the iodine and lemon juice which disinfect, cleanse and fix the tan. This simple product will assure you an even, lovely color and a smooth and supple skin. In tropical lands people use coconut oil and palm oil to guard their skins against the burning sun.

In case of sunburn I advise applying wet dressings saturated in a quince seed solution. Boil four tablespoons of quince core in a quart of water for a quarter of an hour. May I also suggest a tisane which helps the body counter the effects of the burn: one pinch of camomile (the entire plant) and one pinch of lavender to a quart of water. Drink four cups of this per day.

Do not forget the virtues of parsley as a balm for skin irritations and insect bites. Our Lady's Seal helps against bruises, while the daisy is efficacious against swellings. Fresh comfrey root is a remedy for cuts and wounds. The juice of yarrow promotes healing of scratches and sores, while the juice of celandine banishes corns, warts and calluses. For sore feet, add a handful of lavender and a spoonful of salt to a basin of warm water and soak a while.

A famous actress, already elderly but still alluring, asked me for something to firm up her flesh, particularly at the thighs. I recommended a solution made by steeping a pinch of lavender, a pinch of nettles and half a pinch of celandine overnight in a quart of rain water. She used this lotion regularly and thanks to it was able to appear in a bathing suit long after ladies her age would have desisted.

Our hands are an extremely important and expressive part of us and deserve regular care. It is sad to see a pretty woman with unkempt hands. If your skin has become coarsened by heavy labor or much scrubbing, you may quickly undo the damage by rubbing your hands with a lotion made of warm olive oil and a squeeze of lemon juice. This is also good for cracked nails. Lemon by itself is excellent for the hands, whitening and cleansing the skin. Learn to make the most of this fruit; after you have squeezed its juice, rub your hands with the pungent yellow rind. You might also rub your face with it.

Rubbing the hands with vinegar will banish any cooking smells. Coffee grounds absorb garlic odors and fresh parsley neutralizes the smell of onion.

To keep the skin of the chest looking youthful and clear I recommend washing often with tinglingly cold water. You may also rub in almond oil, which helps the skin retain its elasticity. There is also an astringent lotion made by steeping a handful of savory overnight in a quart of water.

From the dawn of time women have been concerned with the beauty of their bodies. Nowadays men, too, have become interested in the matter and are not disposed to let themselves go to seed. The simple recipes I have provided should be as useful to them as to the ladies.

The Face

> *A beautiful face is the finest sight under heaven.*
> —*La Bruyère*

In this belief women have always done everything in their power to improve their faces. Nowadays we have plastic surgery which can correct grave flaws, but when there was no such possibility of reshaping features, women would go to great lengths to preserve the freshness of their complexions.

Over the centuries various forms of skin care have been in vogue. Poppæa, the wife of the emperor Nero who was renowned for her beauty, would apply a mask of rye mash mixed with olive oil. The other ladies of Rome followed suit. Among the Gauls a mixture of chalk moistened with vinegar and the foam of beer was preferred. During the Renaissance a compound of rose petals and curds reigned supreme. In the eighteenth century Mme. Pompadour and the other court ladies would spread thin slices of raw meat on their cheeks to enhance their color. Shortly afterward the fashion of painting the face came in and created such a furor that La Bruyère took note of it, remarking: "If the ladies really possessed the appearance they give themselves by artifice, if they had faces as dazzling as those they make with paints and rouges, they would be inconsolable."

In our own time a succession of products has enjoyed temporary esteem: mink oil, turtle oil, yeast, fish oil and the like. Each was supposed to glorify the skin.

One day I received a visit from a teenage girl and her mother. The girl was strikingly pretty, but her face was covered with dreadful pimples. As her mother explained, this was giving the girl all kinds of complexes. I had first to treat her nerves and then her skin. For the latter I prescribed a lotion made of roses and horsetail. She kept up her cure faithfully and five years later won the title of Miss France. Eventually she married and had a family. She now lives in my part of the country and I see her from time to time. She has remained extremely beautiful and her skin, thanks to the use of my lotion, is still as fresh as roses at sunrise.

A good skin depends on good general health. This involves having sufficient sleep, avoiding stimulants like coffee, alcohol and tobacco, all of which are ruinous to the complexion, and having a liver in sound working order. All the vegetables and herbal teas favorable to sleep and to the digestion will therefore serve you well. I particularly recommend a glass of fruit juice or vegetable juice taken at breakfast. The best vegetable juices are watercress, parsley, celery and cucumber, perhaps with a slice of lemon added.

Then there are depurative teas that clean the system of toxins that might otherwise accumulate and produce blotchings on the nose and chin. Fresh burdock root and the flowers of the wild pansy make highly efficacious drinks. My own special favorite for this purpose is a tea made of wild chicory and bittersweet leaves—one pinch of each of these herbs to a quart of water. This should be drunk at the rate of two cups per day.

The same plants often help the skin externally as well as internally. Burdock, for instance, makes an excellent poultice for all kinds of minor skin troubles from adolescent acne to scurf. Cut a fresh burdock plant and blanch it for a moment in boiling water. Then spread the limp leaves, as hot as possible, over the pimples. If fresh burdock is not available, you may obtain it dried from an herb dealer. Moisten it in boiling water and mix it in equal parts with onion.

Solutions of thyme, sage, rosemary and fennel are all good skin antiseptics. Parsley water, made by steeping a bunch of parsley twenty-four hours in a glass of water, will purify the complexion.

The condition known as roseola, caused by congestion of the capillaries of the face, may either be hereditary or brought on by emotional shocks, as well as sharp changes of temperature. I can suggest a number of decongestive lotions for it. Boil two or three lettuce plants in a saucepan of water and use the liquor as a wash. Another good lotion is made by steeping one pinch of poppy blossoms, one of eglantine, and one of fresh celandine in a quart of spring water. Mallow yields another mild and soothing lotion for roseola and all inflammations of the face. Boil four pinches of mallow blossom for half an hour in a quart of water. The condition, by its nature, is not cleared up in a day, but patient treatment with these lotions will produce happy results.

In general, people's skins are of three kinds: oily, dry and normal. But skin type is really more complicated, for some people have all three kinds of skin at once—for instance, oily skin at the chin, dry skin around the eyes and normal skin on the rest of the face. This naturally complicates the problem of skin care.

Dry skins are the finest in texture but also the most fragile. They very much need oils of some sort. In the absence of fancy creams, you might use ordinary milk as a cleanser and fresh cream as a nutritive.

A massage with simple dairy products of this sort will do you far more good than using creams of doubtful quality. In earlier days women in country districts would even rub their faces with pork fat. This may not seem the daintiest of treatments but it is an effective one.

Once a week you might make up a facial mask by beating the yolk of an egg with a teaspoon of olive oil. Apply this to your face and keep it on for a quarter of an hour, then rinse it away with a wad of cotton dipped in warm milk. For extra-dry skin, add a spoonful of fresh cream to any mask made of fruit or vegetables.

Should wrinkles come, not as a result of age but of dehydration of the skin caused by illness or abrupt loss of weight, you might resort to the following solution: one pinch of wild chicory and one pinch of celandine steeped in a quart of spring water. Bathe your face with this morning and night. The foregoing recipes will also be helpful.

An oily skin is a different proposition. It is generally a problem for young people, since the skin has a tendency to dry out with the years. The important thing is to keep the skin fresh. Frequent washings with warm water will rinse the pores of oil and secretions of sebum. Avoid the use of creams. If you need something for removing makeup, use fresh milk diluted with a few drops of eau de cologne. You may also mix the milk with equal parts of strawberry juice, which soothes and freshens the skin. The aromatic and astringent herbs yield useful lotions: thyme, rosemary, blackberry leaves and hawthorn leaves are all good for this purpose.

Just as the yolk of egg supplies necessary nutrients to dry skins, the white of egg refines the texture of oily skins. You may use it by itself or mixed with fruits and vegetables.

A perfect lotion for dry skins is made in the following manner: steep one pinch of red rose petals, one pinch of sage flowers, one pinch of walnut leaf and one pinch of horsetail overnight in a quart of spring water.

Oily skins are highly susceptible to blackheads. Unsightly and embarrassing as they are, they are not really a serious problem. It is inadvisable to press them out one by one, since that means breaking the skin and inviting infection. In former days the country remedy was to rub the face with quarters of fresh tomato or morsels of ripe pumpkin. Gentle massages of this sort can absorb the imperfections. I have also had good results with an antiblackhead lotion of my own made by steeping one pinch of celandine and one pinch of dandelion root overnight in a quart of spring water.

Even if you are lucky enough to have normal skin, you should take care of it and see to its proper nourishment. Just as your body has to be provided with varied fare comprising proteins, carbohydrates, fats, minerals and vitamins, so your skin needs all these elements. I will not encourage you to lay beefsteaks on your cheeks, as did Mme. Pompadour, but it is a fact that your skin needs meat. Dairy products are also especially welcome. And fruits and vegetables supply the vitamins for which the skin is especially greedy.

Externally, too, fruits and vegetables do wonders for the skin. Today there are numerous beauty products on the market which claim to be made from these, but you can easily make your own with fresh fruit in season. To make the mask more effective, you should take the preliminary step of applying a hot pack to open the pores. Boil up some water with a pinch of linden, or a sprig of thyme, rosemary or sage. Dip a face cloth in this and apply to the face for a few minutes. Then lie down for a quarter of an hour, preferably in the dark, and coat your face with a thin layer of whatever fruit or vegetable you are using, in crushed or grated form. Afterwards wash this mask off with a sponge dipped in warm water.

Among the fruits, the most refreshing masks are made from strawberries, peaches, pineapple and watermelon, either by themselves or washed with a bit of fresh cream or yellow or white of egg, according to the nature of your skin. If you make a grape cure in the autumn and are using lots of grape juice, set aside the skins from the grapes you have been pressing and apply them, fresh, as a mask. Your cure will be that much more thorough.

Among the vegetables, I recommend cucumbers, sliced fine or chopped. They are splendid moisturizers. Grated carrots are good against any inflammation of the face, sunburn or roseola. Carrot juice used as a face lotion will greatly improve the complexion, thanks to its natural coloring matter carotene. It outdoes any amount of makeup.

A mask of chopped cabbage has exceptional virtues. Remember that a cabbage poultice will heal the worst wounds and ulcers. This means that cabbage can absorb impurities and sterilize tissues.

There are those who favor a mask of chopped potatoes, claiming that it moisturizes the skin and banishes wrinkles. Beets, grated and mixed with cream, are said to improve the complexion, while a mask of warm spinach cooked in milk is said to descale the skin.

My general advice is that you divide your dinner between your stomach and your liver, for what is good for one will also be good for the other. You will also, of course, want to eliminate anything harmful to either, such as denatured food and strong stimulants. Alcohol, either internally or externally, has adverse effects upon the skin: cologne water, for instance, dries out the skin. On the other hand, the herbal teas are splendid and you would do well to set aside a half-cup of any tisane you have brewed to use as a wash.

If you want a complexion of lilies and roses, turn to these flowers in your garden. Add a handful of their petals, either fresh or dried, to a pint of boiling water and simmer for a quarter of an hour. Then cool and strain the liquid and pat it gently over your face.

I have male patients, many of whom are actors whose skin is tired from continuous use of makeup. I offer them the same advice that I would to women. For one of the great discoveries of the twentieth century, I think, is that beauty lies within the scope of all, men and women, the poor as well as the rich. And as Rudyard Kipling said: "If you possess beauty and nothing else, God's finest gift is yours."

The Eyes

The eyes are the mirror of the soul, as the saying goes, and we like our mirrors to be brilliant and well polished. The ladies of Andalusia, famous for their fiery glances, put a drop of orange juice into their eyes to make them glisten. Orange juice is less stinging than lemon, and has tonic properties besides.

But a more gentle eye lotion is made from cornflowers, the most azure of all flowers. Country people have long known that corn-flowers are good for the eyes, and not for blue eyes only, though blue eyes are more sensitive than others. A handful of cornflower blossoms is thrown into a pint of boiling water and steeped for a few minutes. The liquid is strained and used as an eyewash. The result is highly refreshing.

Other herbs make good eye disinfectants—plantain, roses, parsley, chervil. A solution of linden applied as a warm compress over the eyes will banish dark circles. Camomile is also good for the eyes though it can produce irritation if used over too long a time. It is better to alternate it with other plants.

I recommend a solution of various herbs, for example one pinch of mallow, one pinch of camomile, two pinches of cornflower and two pinches of either rose or violet petals.

In case of severe conjunctivitis, remember the country legend about celandine. The nightingale is supposed to drop the juice of celandine into the eyes of her nestlings. The ancients, too, considered celandine an eye medicine. However, you should be careful about using this potent but dangerous flower, and I would suggest the following dependable recipe: steep one small pinch of celandine, both flower and stem, plus two or three generous pinches of rose petals overnight in a quart of boiled water. The roses offset whatever strong effect the celandine might have.

Solutions of chervil, parsley or plantain (two or three pinches to a quart of water), may also be cut with rose petals. Solutions of this sort should not be kept longer than a week, because they spoil after a time.

If you wish to keep your eyesight as keen as when you were twenty, eat plenty of blueberries. Remember that they are the favored food of airplane pilots.

The Teeth and Mouth

A radiant smile is one of the qualities most admired in our times. Toothpastes that promise us sparkling teeth and clean breath bring fortunes to their manufacturers. Perfect teeth, in fact, are a mark of youth, and we cannot hope to keep them so forever. However, dentistry has made such progress that we can count on keeping our teeth a good deal longer than our forebears did and there is no longer any excuse for rotten and yellowed teeth.

Dental hygiene should be part of our daily routine. Brushing our teeth morning and night should be a sacred rule. However, there are a few other things we can do to supplement this procedure.

After you have squeezed a lemon, do not discard the precious rind but use it for rubbing over your teeth. This will whiten the teeth and strengthen their roots. An apple munched, peel and all, confers the same benefits, disinfecting the teeth and massaging the gums. I recommend eating an apple in the evening instead of sucking on some sweets—the first is as good for your teeth as the second is bad.

In earlier days people would make an effective dentrifrice from charcoal or burnt toast, mixing the black powder with a few drops of oil of mint. The toothpastes of today have a more agreeable texture, but they, too, usually contain mint, not because of its pleasant flavor but because of its antiseptic qualities. If some irritation of the gums should prevent you from using a toothbrush for a few days, make sure to rinse your mouth with a mint solution.

Such gum infections can be highly painful and rob you of all desire to eat. Make up a mouthwash of mallow, thyme, sage or blackberry leaves and rinse the mouth at hourly intervals with it. You may also rub your gums with lemon juice or onion juice. Very soon you will be able to smile again.

When children have difficulty teething, give them the root of mallow to chew on. Older people whose teeth are getting shaky might try chewing slowly on a bit of horseradish.

The Hair

In the past, a woman's long, flowing hair used to be considered one of her glories. In the twenties this changed and no chic woman wanted to have long hair. In recent years the fashion has reversed and girls once more pride themselves on their rich manes. But whether cropped or flowing, the condition of the hair has always had an important bearing on a woman's appearance.

The hairdressers' salons contain a regular arsenal of beauty: all sorts of shampoos, lotions, tints and sprays. There are chemicals for smoothing too wild curls and others for putting waves into the straightest of locks. But can any of these products bring health to the hair? More likely they do the opposite.

When I was a child I used to enjoy watching the womenfolk of my family looking after their hair. In this matter they were guided by customs and traditions. Thus it was a rule among them that hair must never be cut except at the time of the new moon; otherwise you might injure its delicate fiber and stop it from growing. Washing the hair was a solemn act in those days. At other times the women might undo their ample buns and let their hair come tumbling down over their shoulders. Then they would sit and slowly rub their scalps with olive oil to nourish the hair roots. They would wrap their heads in warm towels and let the oil work for several hours.

If someone's hair were too oily, she made up a shampoo of eggs and rum—two yolks of eggs beaten up with a shot glass of rum. She would apply this mixture, the color of sunlight, and let it stay on for a good quarter of an hour.

After the shampoo women would rinse their hair with a dash of vinegar. This gave a sheen to their hair. Or if someone wanted her hair to be especially silky, she would rinse it with a solution of burdock root.

To alter their hair color they would use a solution of camomile, which is a gentle bleach and gives the hair a lovely golden luster. Or else they might use strong tea, which imparts a russet tint to the hair.

Why not revive some of these old-fashioned procedures? These herbal ingredients are easier to use than complicated chemicals and have no harmful side effects. You might even try bypassing commercial shampoos and using soapwort (or bouncing bet), that common roadside flower with pale pink blossoms that in the past was prized as a cleanser of delicate fabrics. During the war, when regular soaps were unavailable in France, an extract was made from this plant which served as an effective laundry detergent. Pull up some soapwort and chop its roots. Throw a generous handful of these roots into a quart of boiling water, let it steep for ten minutes, strain and use as a shampoo. You will find that your hair emerges clean, silky and healthy from this bath.

Many men feel it is a tragedy to lose their hair. They think baldness is a sort of disgrace. They should know that they may insure themselves against this danger by making a practice of drinking a small glass of watercress juice at breakfast. The same watercress juice acts as an effective tonic when rubbed into the scalp. Another excellent hair tonic is based on nasturtium. The recipe for this may be found in Chapter 4. Still another remedy against baldness is the following: Steep one pinch of nettle flower, one of sage blossom, one pinch of burdock (using the entire plant) and one pinch of bay leaf in a quart of water. Let the mixture stand for twenty-four hours. Wet your hair generously with this solution.

We now come to the question of perfume and scents. In the past these would be made up in the home. Since there are so many commercial types on the market today, no one thinks of compounding her own personal fragrance. Yet the process is easy enough.

To make a lavender water you have only to steep 25 grams of the flower in a quart of alcohol. Let it stand for a month, strain it and bottle it for year-round use. You might gather the flowers during your vacation trip. Such lavender water is equally appreciated by men and women and is useful not only as a perfume but as a body rub and remedy against rheumatism.

In much the same fashion you can prepare toilet waters of rose, jasmine, violet, citronella and all the herbs and flowers whose fragrance you especially enjoy. You might try verbena, mint, thyme, rosemary.

At the beginning of the eighteenth century a perfume-maker of Cologne, Jean-Marie Farina, compounded a toilet water which has made his name immortal. This is the eau de Cologne which is popular to this day. You can make one very much like it in the following fashion: Heat a quart of alcohol. Add 4 grams each of the following essences: orange blossom oil, oil of rosemary, oil of cedar and oil of bergamot. Let stand twenty-four hours and bottle.

Over the centuries many perfumes have been devised for the purpose of seduction. These have been popular with men as well as with women. Some became famous in their time and were given high-sounding names. Thus we have had the Perfume of the Crusades (lavender, marjoram, basil, savory, rosemary), the Bouquet of the Empress Eugénie (rose, vanilla, geranium) and the Perfume of the Queen of England (rose, violet, orange blossom). Some more frankly aphrodisiac were given such names as the Perfume of Wild Kisses (citronella, verbena, jonquil, musk and ambergris) or in a more pastoral vein, Bouquet of New-Mown Hay.

I take pleasure in the knowledge that through all the ages my friends the plants have been mankind's best allies in the quest for beauty and love.

7. Tell Me What You Eat

Animals feed, men eat. But only the cultivated man knows the art of eating.

So wrote Brillat-Savarin, whose *The Physiology of Taste* is at once a work on philosophy and cooking. I heartily agree with him. I, too, think that we need considerable intelligence and sensitivity to nourish ourselves properly.

I am against those rigid and unimaginative diets which limit our choices in the realm of food. Such diets may be healthful but they undermine our pleasure in life. In the case of illness, to be sure, a strict diet must be followed, but in general we must above all have variety. Though I have spent many pages stressing the importance of vegetables and herbs, I would not want to be taken for a fanatical vegetarian or an advocate of spartan living. On the contrary. I have all the normal appetites, including a liking for good food. I love the good things of this earth too well to become a preacher of abstinence.

At the risk of shocking some nutrition extremists, I would say that it is better to sit down to a slice of *foie gras* from a goose raised on pure grain than to a soup of leeks raised with chemical fertilizer. Yet people persist in thinking that they are doing themselves all sorts of good by going on a strict diet. Here, I would say, is another case of good intentions going astray. For nature presents a picture of variety; what we eat should also be varied. Vegetables are an important component in our diet, but we need animal food as well. In our times the general level of nutrition in the developed countries has risen greatly, with a consequent improvement in general health and longevity. I would not wish to see us return to the spartan fare of poor peasants of the past, who had to do a hard day's labor on an onion and a heel of bread. Yet I cannot approve of the gluttonous banquets in which the privileged classes indulge.

Our eating pattern should fall midway between these two extremes and should be neither too rich nor too scanty. The one requirement I feel strongly about is the quality of our food-stuffs. I would like to see us all making our choice on this basis. An honest food product has nothing to hide. The processor should be able to frankly state what has gone into it. The consumer should be able to know what he is buying and pass up any product about which he has doubts. With the problem of quality out of the way, there remains only the matter of shaping the family menu so that it is both tasty and healthful.

Just as we have made a careful study of each vegetable, fruit and aromatic herb that figures in our diet, so we should be aware of the properties of every kind of meat, fish, dessert and drink that appears on our table. Nutrition is not a matter of blind chance. We have the saying: "Tell me what you eat and I'll tell you what you are." There is more medical truth to this adage than you may think. People who eat a good deal of meat are energetic and dynamic, but if they go too far in this direction they become highly aggressive, and with the passing years they manifest typical physiologic disturbances such as an excess of cholesterol and uric acid, which lead to arteriosclerosis and gout. People who are too fond of carbohydrates and sweets will be overweight and have a tendency toward diabetes. As for the vegetarian, though he is generally considered to be eating wisely, he will be something of a weakling and wears his body out too soon by cheating it of necessary proteins.

Man is by nature, I am convinced, omnivorous. In the earliest stages of his evolution he subsisted by gathering roots, leaves and fruits, but also by hunting and fishing. Everywhere in the world and among the most primitive people we find a similar pattern. African natives hunt big game. But they also raise various tubers and fruits, and supplement their diet with insects and berries. In those parts of the world where vegetation is scarce, as for example in Lapland, the natives have learned to use whatever tiny plants they can find, even mosses and lichens. The same is true in desert regions.

Children should therefore be taught from the earliest age to eat a miscellany of food. Evidence shows that the early nutritional pattern exerts a determining influence on an individual's future health and intelligence. Hence our contemporary practice of introducing infants of only a few weeks to a wide variety of foods rich in proteins, vitamins and minerals. Babies are no longer fed only on milk and porridge. They are given fruit juice, strained vegetables, fish and meats along with their bottles. They savor a bit of cheese long before they have any teeth. The result is that they are more alert, better-humored and quicker to walk than they used to be.

The child-care books of a previous day would advise mothers to provide one kind of diet for boy children and another for girls. Boys were supposed to be given stimulating and dynamic foods like meats, fish and eggs, with perhaps a bit of wine now and then. Girls, on the other hand, were supposed to be given sweets, custards and pastries, which would, it was thought, prolong their years of childish innocence. All that is long since out of style, and the modern girl prefers a rare steak to a cream puff.

Adults, however, are in another boat and commit many nutritional errors out of laziness. The average man, condemned to taking a quick lunch at a cafeteria, will choose the same menu practically every day: some sort of hors d'oeuvre, steak and fried potatoes, or chicken and fried potatoes, and a piece of cheese, or some sort of cake. The result is that he is subsisting on heavy, concentrated foods, high in fats and low in vitamins. Eating this way all year around, year after year, deprives his body of the variety of elements so essential to good health.

The sensible housewife, will offer her family on ever-changing array of foods to keep their vitality at its peak. A considerable proportion of this menu will be fruits and vegetables. I myself am a great believer in the single-course dinner combining a multiplicity of elements. Consider, for example, the chicken stew for which Gascony is famous. Our good King Henri IV, who knew a thing or two about nutrition, wanted this to be the universal Sunday dish throughout his realm. It would contain, first of all, a hen, an old and somewhat tough one whose laying days were over. This would have put the dish within the reach of even the poorest peasants. Nowadays the fact that a hen has lived a long and useful life scratching about in the yard is a sign of quality. Properly treated, such a fowl is a good deal tastier than a mass-produced broiler. To make up for the dryness of older chicken, you will want to put some chopped bacon or fatty sausage meat into the stuffing. Also included will be some eggs, which add protein to the dish, bread soaked in milk and a handful of aromatic herbs (garlic, onion, parsley, thyme, rosemary, etc.), which contribute their special properties. The stuffed chicken is set to boil with an assortment of vegetables rich in vitamins and minerals. As a result, even a small portion of this chicken stew gives you all that you need for healthful eating.

There are many other ways to bring variety to the table without resorting to complicated menus. Soups of mixed vegetables are excellent and so is every sort of stew. There are also the mixed salads, which contain a profusion of fresh vegetables all thrown in together and garnished with chopped herbs. You might also serve desserts consisting of fruit salad containing all the available fruits of the season and sprinkled with prunes, raisins and chopped nuts.

A splendid treat for children is the so-called mendicant, which takes its name from the four mendicant orders, the Dominicans, the Augustines, the Franciscans and the Carmelites. Vowed to frugality and asceticism, these orders would allow themselves only those dried fruits like figs, raisins, hazelnuts and almonds whose brown skin matched their own brown habits. But give a child a handful of these natural goodies and he will be content, as well as excellently nourished.

Of all the jams the best one in my opinion is the good old-fashioned *raisiné*, whose recipe you will find in Chapter 8. It includes a large variety of vegetables and fruit and is entirely free of artificial ingredients like refined sugar. Spread on a good slice of bread, it makes an ideal snack for a child.

To be sure, all these counsels only apply to meals eaten at home. In this respect they run counter to modern life, where even children take their meals at the school lunchroom. Yet this necessity only underlines the importance of what is served at the family table, since the family meal has to make up for the deficiencies of the others.

There have been some among my patients who, convinced of

the necessity of having a balanced diet, have been willing to
ch____ge their pattern of life, and even give up their practice of
____ business lunches. They report that they feel far better since
_____ The most thoroughgoing of these is the singer Marcel
_____ ecause of his profession he was always on tour and
_____ t hotels and take his meals more or less at random.
_____ e when his health broke down and I helped him
_____ s of a strict diet. When he was well again and
_____ avels, he bought himself a trailer and hired a
h_____ _____ for him. Now he is able to eat properly
wh___ _____ elf, and as a result can continue with his
caree_ _____ st amount of energy his profession requires \ _____ medicines. Nowadays I regard him
not so m___ _____ friend and I have immense respect
for his stren___ _____ high professional standards.

But now le___ _____ r gastronomy rather than of nutrition. It
is certainly a m___ ____eerful approach to the problem of eating and
we need not lose any of the benefits to our health and happiness
thereby.

Meats

Vegetarians have presented a great many arguments in their
effort to stem the enormous consumption of meat that goes on
all over the world. Their first argument is a moral one: that it
is horrible to kill animals to eat their flesh. They have also put
forth various medical arguments, contending that meat is difficult
to digest and produces wastes and fermentations that poison
the organism. They have even turned for support to anthropology,
and point out that the human molar differs markedly from the
molar of carniverous species, and that human canine teeth are
meant not for tearing meat but for cracking nuts.

Their efforts are in vain. As a country grows more prosperous,
its consumption of meat rises. And the health of the people
seems to follow the same curve. The fact is that meat is richer
than any other food in energy-giving protein.

I myself favor beef and lamb over all the other meats, not so much because these are more nutritious as because they are less apt to be contaminated by chemical additives. Cattle and sheep pasture on grass, their natural food, while calves raised for veal and pigs raised by large-scale methods, as most of them are, are plied with various feeds containing a significant admixture of hormones and antibiotics. I have already discussed the dangers of this kind of feeding in Chapter 1. This has become so serious a matter that I would suggest that you do not buy these meats except from a dependable butcher who can vouch for the quality of his wares.

The way in which meat is cooked is also of great importance. I do not approve of steak tartare or extremely rare steaks. Meat has to be cooked long enough to destroy whatever microbes may be present. This is especially true of pork.

Today the preferred way to treat meat is to grill it, and this is healthier than frying. However, you should keep in mind that a marbleized steak is actually streaked through and through with fat, and that this fat does not disappear even after grilling. Thus you are eating sheer cholesterol. You should therefore trim away as much of the fat as you can. The same is true of stew meat or pot roast. A tablespoon of olive oil at the bottom of your casserole is far less harmful than a morsel of animal fat. In general, vegetable fats are far less dangerous than animal fats. Should your roast seem too dry, you might add a bit of butter or a dash of olive oil to it after it has been cooked to improve its savor.

Sausage meats are often high in indigestible fats and have been doctored with chemicals and artificial coloring matter. One well-known trick is to disguise pork fat by tinting it pink. Those fine plump sausages you trustfully buy will cook down to half their size; in truth, there is almost no real meat in them. If you must have sausages, try to buy them direct from some farmer. A home-raised pig has been fed on skim-milk, surplus vegetables and kitchen scraps; it has led an energetic life and will taste quite different from the indolent, commercially raised hog. In the past the family pig would supply the farmer with his whole year's quota of meat and no part of the animal was permitted to go to waste. The country saying used to be: "With a pig, you use everything except the squeak"—and this was true. Black pudding, sausage meat, salami, hams, chops, *pâtés, rillettes,* roasts, tripe, lard —all of these can be valuable foods if used in moderation. The frugal peasant made a meal of a bit of smoked bacon and heavy bread and this did him no harm because both the bread and the pork were natural products.

Poultry and game make excellent eating, though I must again put in a word for moderation and some assurance as to quality. Rabbit and hare are low in fat and therefore are recommended for those who must be careful about their weight or their cholestorol count. Moreover, rabbit is among the least expensive meats.

Many people have sworn off chicken ever since the scandal of the hormones used in poultry feed was widely publicized. But rather than rule out chicken altogether, it makes more sense to set certain standards of quality. Every food has its justification. In the United States, where a great deal of turkey is eaten, scientists have discovered that turkey meat has definite benefits for people with arthritis and psoriasis. In fact, turkey meat must be regarded as medicinal!

As a closing word, let me say something about *foie gras,* that most elegant and also most condemned of all meat products. To be sure, it is not a light dish. It should be saved for some little celebration, when we feel we want to partake of something special. Under such circumstances a bit of *foie gras* rejoices the heart and therefore promotes digestion. We should not deny ourselves this gastronomic delight altogether because of its high fat content, or eat it with so much guilt that we soon feel sick to our stomach. *Foie gras* has an illustrious history. It was discovered by the Greeks, who fattened their geese by feeding them with pellets of wheat moistened in water. The Romans improved on this method by adding dry figs to the feed they gave their geese. Extremely partial to the liver of their geese, they named the dish made of that liver *ficatum*—or "fed on figs." Curiously enough, etymologists tell us, this word became the root of the French word for liver: *foie.* Thus the term used in cooking came to designate the organ. Here is an interesting example of culinary knowledge antedating anatomical knowledge. It seems proper, then, that this dish with its long historical associations should remain in our cookbooks and on our tables—for very special occasions.

Seafood

Not too long ago people did penance on Friday by eating fish rather than meat. This Catholic custom had one distinct advantage from a nutritional standpoint: people were forced to eat fish at least once a week. It meant, furthermore, that on Fridays the fish shops were well supplied and housewives could find an abundant choice even in the smallest towns at great distance from the sea.

Today fish is available the week round and everywhere. Advances in transport and in refrigeration techniques have made this possible.

But even though Friday is no longer an official fast day, it is still a good idea to introduce fish into the family diet at least once a week. Ocean fish are rich in iodine and chlorine, while freshwater fish contain potassium, magnesium and phosphorous. The various forms of seafood have an exceptionally high vitamin content. Oysters, especially, are rich in iodine and improve the circulation.

Unfortunately, our rivers, and now the oceans, have been ravaged by pollution. A worldwide effort must be made to save them. For if the weary earth can no longer feed its children, the oceans hold riches we may still draw upon.

Bread and Cereals

Is bread sacred or accursed? That is a perplexing question. From earliest times bread has been a symbol of God's gift of life to man. Jesus performed a miracle with bread, so that a single loaf could feed a multitude, and men break bread together as a sign of friendship and sharing. But in our own days bread has become something of a menace.

The Lord's Prayer says: "Give us this day our daily bread." But nowadays sophisticated people look away from the bread basket with disgust and say: "Thank you, I never eat bread." In France bread consumption has fallen off by half in the past fifty years. This may be the sign of prosperity and a varied diet. But it is also a sign of repudiation.

The white bread we see in our bakeries has lost almost all of its vitamins, its proteins, its phosphates, its calcium, its amino acids. For all these precious elements are contained in the husk and the germ of the wheat, and are discarded in the milling of white flour. All that remains is starch—a lifeless component, best used for fattening hogs. The worst of this is that the government has had a decisive role in the matter. The French government regulates the amount of wheat grown and sets standards for the treatment of the grain. When the crop is plentiful and the wheat harvest exceeds the government's quota, a lower percentage of flour is extracted—65 percent, for example; the figure is adjusted from year to year. If, on the other hand, the crop is smaller than expected, more of the grain is utilized. Thus we arrive at the paradox that we may be supplied with a far better bread in times of hardship and war than in times of peace and plenty. In point of fact, this is not so, for the whole wheat of wartime bread was stretched by so many ersatz ingredients that the bread was scarcely more digestible than plaster. All of this is done entirely without the consent of the consumer. Of all the foods we eat, we have the least control over that which should be the cornerstone of our diet—bread.

Other misfortunes have befallen bread. With the rigid control of working hours, bakers and their assistants must turn out larger quantities of bread within a shorter time span. This has led to the development of various artificial rising agents that work faster than good, old-fashioned yeast. To make matters worse, electric ovens have replaced the old wood-fired ones.

Such developments proceed inexorably to the point where bread loses not only its nutritive properties but even its taste. The nadir has been reached in the United States, where the bread is truly no longer fit to eat. The gradual abandonment of bread in France may be seen as a warning signal. In fact, only such quiet and prolonged boycotts will force those entrusted with the production of bread to reverse their course.

Fortunately, there are some bakeries turning out so-called country bread made of whole wheat and rye flours, costing somewhat more but considerably more filling and satisfying. These I recommend unreservedly, so long as they are honest products made without fraud. To deserve the name of country bread, it must be made with real yeast and baked in a wood-fired oven. It should be truly made of whole grains, not of white flour to which some bran has been added. Such whole-grain breads are rich in many vitamins. Rye bread, moreover, is gently laxative.

Unground wheat, still in its kernel, is a rare commodity these days. That is a pity, because it is a tasty and healthful cereal, a veritable food in itself. I would like to see it available in groceries along with rice. Those who live in country districts, however, can easily supply themselves with wheat. Let me suggest that they try eating wheat sprouts, which are extremely rich in vitamin C. This is how to go about sprouting your wheat: Put a handful of wheat in a bowl of water. Let it soak for two days. Then rinse the wheat carefully and lay it out on a plate. The next day, wash the wheat again. Soon a little white sprout appears. It is well to wash your wheat still another time before you eat it. The sprouts may be used either raw in a salad or cooked in soups, stews and pancakes. Use it with moderation, for it is a very rich food.

Among the other cereals, I recommend cornmeal, which is highly nourishing and easy to digest. In southern France and in Italy it is greatly appreciated and used in *polenta* and other tasty dishes. Oats, on the other hand, are associated more with northern lands where breakfast porridge forms a staple of the diet. With its unique texture, oatmeal is especially good for diabetics, who are otherwise restricted in their use of cereals and starches.

Barley, particularly used in broth, promotes calcification. Rye is laxative and prevents arteriosclerosis. In countries like Russia and Poland, where rye bread is the staff of life, there is very little incidence of cardiovascular disturbances. As for buckwheat, which we use largely in pancakes, it helps strengthen the blood vessels. On this score alone it should be more widely used.

Dairy Products

We have long been told that milk is the ideal food for children. It is considered the most healthful of all foods. On the other hand, it is highly susceptible to spoilage, is the perfect culture medium for microbes of every sort and carries whatever toxins the cow may have absorbed.

Pasteurization, to be sure, was a remarkable discovery, and since Dr. Pasteur was a Frenchman, it accrues to our national glory. Nevertheless, it does not provide an infallible guarantee of purity. Certain viruses are resistant to heat.

Moreover, many milk producers neglect the ordinary rules of sanitation, with the excuse that, after all, the milk is going to be pasteurized. Dirty barns and dirty milk utensils are too often the rule. In fact, some have said that pasteurization has become a permit for filth.

Meanwhile the housewife, reassured by the label "pasteurized" on her carton of milk, no longer takes the trouble to scald it as she used to in the past. Let me take this opportunity to suggest that milk should be treated with the greatest care, particularly when fed to a child. It is a healthful food when it is perfectly sanitary. Should its cleanliness be the least doubtful, or should it have begun to sour, you had best throw it away.

Some adults maintain that they cannot tolerate milk. In fact, even the purest milk is indigestible for certain people. Mixed with coffee, as in our traditignal French *café au lait,* it can be even worse—a veritable poison for the liver. The best way to take milk is in cooked form, in creamed soups or custards. Newborn babies used to be given milk mixed with barley water. The addition of the barley made the milk more digestible, almost like mother's milk.

Milk is an excellent antidote against many poisons. Should a child eat something dangerous, give it great quantities of milk to drink while waiting for the doctor.

Junket and yogurt are both excellent sources of lactic acid. The natives of Bulgaria, famous for their longevity, are said to owe their health to the daily consumption of yogurt. Nevertheless, a word of warning is in order. The acids of yogurt rob the body of calcium. Here is another food that should not be eaten in excess.

Nowadays the stores carry a great number of milk desserts tricked out with artificial color and flavors. I do not recommend them. Scientists have become suspicious about the use of coloring matter in food; it is a possible cause of cancer. When in doubt, it is always better to abstain. Serve your children unflavored yogurt, cottage cheese and simple milk puddings to which you yourself may add some safe flavoring like chocolate syrup, vanilla or wholesome jam.

Finally there is cheese, an important source of protein. In France we divide cheese into two categories: the cooked and the uncooked. The latter are not fermented and are easier to digest. But keep in mind their fat content. If you are concerned about your weight and your cholesterol count, you must not throw caution to the winds when you are offered the platter of cheeses. One sliver is all you may have. Very well! Savor it.

Sweets

For ages and ages men made do with the natural sugars present in fruits and vegetables. Our sweet tooth was considerably less developed. It was not until the Napoleonic era that sugar began to be extracted on a large scale from sugar beets: a remarkable advance, but not exactly a blessed one.

I have much the same attitude toward refined sugar as I have toward white flour—highly negative. Like white flour, sugar is a lifeless substance, high in calories and low in vitamins. Brown sugar extracted from sugar cane is somewhat less pernicious.

But we have among us some tireless laborers who, according to a secret process known to them alone, are continually engaged in making sugar that is both rich and fragrant: I mean, of course, the bees.

In antiquity it was assumed that honey was one of the prime foods of the gods. Everywhere on earth it has always been considered among the noblest of foods. The Koran, for instance, teaches that the disappearance of honey would be Allah's punishment of men: "The first good that God will take from man will be honey."

But for the moment, Allah be thanked, honey is still available. Let us make the most of it. It contains various forms of sugar that are energy-giving and easy to digest, mineral salts and formic acid, the bee's own chemical additive which insures the honey against spoilage and endows it with certain antibacterial qualities. Hence I recommend adding honey to desserts and thereby disinfecting the digestive and intestinal tract. Honey added to drinks will do the same for the throat and chest, particularly in case of sore throat or tonsillitis.

Honey is good for children, even for very young children. But they should not have too much of it, for it is laxative.

The best honey is undoubtedly made in mountainous regions where the bees graze on remote meadows far from the smoke of factories, the exhausts of autos and the drift of insecticides. This natural honey is far superior to the honey produced by large-scale methods, where the bees are provided with the leftover products of sugar refineries. On the other hand, the beekeeper who sees that his bees have access to aromatic herbs like thyme, rosemary and marjoram, to fields of clover or avenues of linden, will have some wonderful honey to show for his pains. If you live in the country, by all means keep a hive or two of your own.

An interesting medical point: in addition to its own virtues, honey will contain those of the flowers on which the bees have browsed. Thus honey made from linden blossom will be calming, while the honey made from rosemary will be stimulating. Thyme honey has a disinfectant effect on the bronchi, while heather honey benefits the urinary system.

Make a point, then, of having a jar of honey in your cupboard— as a food, a medicament and a taste treat.

Jams, like honey, incorporate the virtues of the fruits and berries from which they have been made. Avoid commercial jams manufactured with artificial flavors and coloring matter. Look for those labeled "made with pure fruit." If you can cook up your own jams and jellies, by all means do so. For sweetening, you may use honey or the juice of grape. (See the recipe for *"raisiné"* in Chapter 8.) Jams may be either laxative or the opposite, as I have explained in connection with blueberries, quinces, prunes and rhubarb.

Chocolate and candy, which children are so fond of, should be eaten only in small quantities, for they put a strain on the liver and spoil the teeth. If you want to give a child something sweet and energy-enhancing, offer him some dried fruits like figs, apricots, raisins, or else a well-ripened banana. Natural candies made with honey are also available.

Where cakes are concerned, the simple ones are always preferable. Should the choice be between a good fruit pie made at home and an elaborate creation of the pastry-maker's covered with artificially tinted frostings and fancy creams, the answer is self-evident. Pass by the tempting window of the pastry shop.

Beverages

What should we drink? First and foremost, we should drink water, that most natural of thirst-quenchers. Since two-thirds of our body weight consists of water, we obviously need to drink. People can survive long fasts and severe hunger, but the absence of water leads very quickly to death.

Even more alarming than the threat of worldwide famine is the possibility of a scarcity of drinkable water. Scientists are already studying techniques for desalinating ocean water. Meanwhile, it is of utmost importance that we look after our rivers, so many of which are already polluted. Even spring water is apt to be polluted by the insecticides with which the ground is saturated.

We drink a great deal of wine in France, sometimes with the excuse that alcohol kills germs. That is to some degree true, and that is why I recommend drinking grog to fend off the grippe. Nevertheless, though I am from Gascony, which prides itself on its vines, I myself drink sparingly. I have learned over the years to prefer quality to quantity. I do not condone that daily quart of coarse red wine with which so many Frenchmen like to wash down their meals, nor that succession of *apértifs* and sweet liqueurs tossed down at the bistro. All these cheap adulterated wines poison the system. Drunk in quantity, they lead all too soon to cirrhosis of the liver.

On the other hand, a single bottle of good wine, by preference red, for it is more easily assimilated than white wine, makes a happy addition to those little parties we sometimes permit ourselves. Let your watchword be: "A little, but of the best." You should not balk at the price of a superior wine. The label saying: "Bottled at the Château" is your assurance of high quality. Drink it slowly and savor every sip.

Though I am strongly opposed to giving wine to children, I recommend it for the aged. In the past old people used to regale themselves with a biscuit or a slice of bread dipped in a half-glass of wine. This was an excellent pick-me-up.

Considered as a tonic, wine has its virtues. But its effectiveness depends on restricted use. Athletes must keep away from it: wine spoils their form. As for lovers who hope that wine will increase their raptures, they will find that it may temporarily inspire them, but if they turn to it regularly, it will in the long run weaken their sexual powers. The reputation of wine as an aphrodisiac is highly questionable.

The same is true of other alcoholic drinks. They are good in limited amounts, dangerous in quantity. As an example, let me cite the armagnac for which my region is famed. It is probably the oldest distilled liquor, the process having been discovered in 1285 by Arnaud de Villeneuve, a celebrated alchemist and physician to the Pope. Yet the distilled spirit was used exclusively as a medicinal product, not as an accompaniment to the pleasures of life.

Probably it was not until the time of Henri IV that the court came to be familiar with the wider uses of this medicine. No doubt it was found to raise the morale of the troops through the long years of warfare that brought Henri to the throne of France. And five centuries later the American writer Hemingway, describing the assualt on Paris by the troops of the Resisance, pays tribute to the part played by armagnac in that historic episode:

> The day we advanced on Paris it rained heavily and everyone was soaked to the skin within an hour of leaving Rambouillet. We proceeded through Chevreuse and St. Rémy-lès-Chevreuse where we had formerly run patrols and were well known to the local inhabitants, from whom we had collected information and with whom we had downed considerable quantities of armagnac to still the ever-present discontent of our guerrillas who were

very Paris-conscious at this time. In those days I had found that
the production of an excellent bottle of any sort of alcholic
beverage was the only way of ending an argument.

Occasions of this sort seem to me the appropriate ones for
alcohol—but such occasions come seldom.

Another drink with a long history is coffee. It was first adopted
in clubs or coffeehouses frequented by the better people. Nowadays cafés are everywhere and coffee-drinking has become thoroughly democratized. The danger is that people drink coffee to
excess. We should remember that coffee is a drug. It is all right
to have a cup when we need to feel particularly stimulated. But
if we drink it every day, and at the rate of several cups at a
time, it will affect the heart. I feel it is very important that we
exercise care concerning the stimulants (alcohol, coffee, tobacco)
that have come to be taken for granted as part of our daily life.

Tea, though considerably lighter than coffee, also can affect
the heart. Nevertheless, it is a good diuretic and may be safely
drunk if you become accustomed to a very light brew, with just
enough tea leaves to perfume the water. The subtle taste is very
enjoyable.

I have already said a great deal about various tisanes and
their medicinal properties. But you may want to invent your
own beverages, for there is no limit to what you may use,
whether fruit, vegetable, herb or grain. In wartime the popular
imagination creates all kinds of substitutes, many of which deserve to be perpetuated. In France we recall the drinks made of
roasted barley, of wheat, of soy beans or chick peas to take the
place of coffee. An interesting drink was made of grated carrots,
which should not be so surprising since carrots are in the same
family as chicory. Roasted, the roots strongly resemble each other
in taste.

In place of their missing tea people concocted substitutes from
sage and blackberry leaves. Why not continue drinking these,
since they have medicinal virtues?

In addition, it used to be a French custom for each household to make up its own liqueurs and light wines of whatever
small fruits were handy. This included mulberry, blueberry,
wild plum, elderberries, chokecherries. Drinks of this sort would
provide an important source of vitamins throughout the win-

ter. Nowadays we can buy canned and bottled fruit juices all year around. These are far preferable from the health standpoint to fruit-flavored sodas. Of course, it is better still to drink the juice of fresh fruits in season. For this is the very lifeblood of the trees, drawn from the soil and ripened by the generous sun.

My purpose in writing this chapter on food in general is to point out the many alternatives we have in this matter of nourishing ourselves. Just as landscape is divided into meadows, orchards, forests, so we should divide our diet between the different branches of food, all healthful and delicious, all the gifts of the earth.

8. A Sheaf of Favorite Recipes

I am neither a master chef nor a gourmet, only a plant-healer who likes to eat. To my mind, the art of cooking consists of preparing meals that are uncomplicated, healthful and appetizing.

I have therefore made a selection of recipes that illustrate these virtues. Some of the dishes feature my favorite plants. Others are traditional recipes, long cherished in my part of the world. Still others have been suggested by my family and friends. I have often been a guest at their tables and in their kindness they have tried to please my tastes. I can testify that I find every dinner with them a feast, with each dish as delicious as it is simple.

I have also had the good fortune to know some real artists in the field of gastronomy, like Raymond Olivier. He has been kind enough to place at my disposal the remarkable collection of old cookery books he has assembled at his home in Bourdonne near Montfort-l'Aumary. Many of these ancient books on gastronomy are rare enough to belong in a museum. Browsing through them is an enlightening experience. I have come across some fantastic recipes in their pages, as well as much sensible advice on domestic economy.

If you own some old cookbooks belonging to your grandmother, do not throw them away. Take time to look through them. You will find a wealth of good sense there and considerable humor besides. Merely reading some of their recipes, you will start to salivate, and that is a good sign. Why not try preparing a good soup according to the book's directions? What comforted men's stomachs and hearts two generations ago can still do so today.

I offer these recipes in a simplified form, for I assume that the mistress of your house knows the basic rules for cooking a stew or a roast. I feel I can trust her discretion in the matter of quantities and proportions. Thus when I say a handful or a pinch, she will know pretty well what I mean.

These recipes are merely suggestions and by no means exhaust the possibilities of the various fruits and vegetables mentioned. When I include a carrot jam to please the children, I am not ruling out the innumerable other things you can do with carrots, from grated carrot salad to carrots in cream sauce, from carrots sautéed with garlic and parsley to carrots included in a stew.

These recipes are for the most part aimed at people in good health. It goes without saying that diabetics must do without jams, and people with heart disease without rich sauces. I am torn between the desire to include various recipes for ragouts and rich sauces and the modern preference for simple grilled meat. Those aromatic herbs whose virtues I preach would go so beautifully into sauces! I sometimes have a hard time reconciling these opposed principles.

If your health permits it, allow yourself an occasional little feast in which you indulge in some of these forbidden delights. Of course, you will want to include some digestive herb like parsley in these rich dishes, and drink a cup of mint tea afterwards. You may also finish the dinner off with a little glass of some homemade liqueur. That will render the rich food harmless.

But most of the time, keep to simple cooking. The recipes I offer are very sensible, and these herb soups and fresh salads will prove to you that eating healthfully is not a penance. There are happy dishes, as there are happy individuals, and these are not always the costliest or the richest.

Remember that at your table no dishes take precedence over others and none are treated as poor relations. The nettles of the field are the equal of asparagus.

Soups

Garlic Soup

In Gascony this is considered the poor man's soup, but it might also grace the table of a king, for it is particularly tasty. What is more, the housewife can prepare it in a few moments. Our grandmothers used to make this soup on the days when they were working in the fields and did not have time to fix their usual cabbage soup, which requires long simmering.

Cut up six or seven plump cloves of garlic and set these to fry in some olive oil. Be careful not to let them burn, for garlic browns quickly. Now add a quart of water or, if you have it, some vegetable, chicken or beef stock. Let this come to a boil for a few moments, then lower the heat. Separate one or two eggs. Add first the white to the hot liquid, stirring energetically, then add the yellow, which you have mixed with two tablespoons of vinegar. Add salt and pepper and serve with croutons.

The same soup can be made with onions and with tomato, or with both of these together. The additional vegetables are cut up and browned along with the garlic. But the key factor is always the garlic.

Aïgo Bouïdo

The name of this soup means *boiled water*, but if the broth is clear, it is nevertheless very savory. It is a great favorite in Provence and is the cousin of our Gascon garlic soup.

Pour some olive oil into the bottom of your soup pot. Add a half-dozen good cloves of garlic chopped coarsely. Since you are eating Provençal style, you will also want to throw in a handful of dry herbs—thyme, fennel, a sprig of sage and a few bay leaves.

Add a quart of water and let the mixture boil at least a quarter of an hour, so that the herbs may give up their full fragrance. Then you will want to strain the mixture, or your family will be bothered by all the bits of dried herbs that get between the teeth. The final step is to add some eggs, as was done in the garlic soup. Pour the soup into an earthenware tureen: its fragrance will perfume the entire dining room.

In Provence this soup is sometimes made with fish. Cut some fish fillets into strips and add to the pot at the same time that you add the water. This does not add appreciably to the cooking time or to the cost and makes the soup an epicure's delight.

Creamed Onion Soup

This is a good soup for those who are less than enthusiastic about the taste of onion, since the milk tempers that taste considerably.

Chop two onions and set them to fry in butter over gentle heat. When they are barely golden, add a pint of milk and let it slowly come to a boil. Remove from the stove and add the yolks of two eggs. Season with salt and pepper and serve with croutons or slices of toasted bread.

Creamed Garlic Soup

This is made exactly the same way as the onion soup, except that garlic takes the place of the onion and olive oil the place of the butter. The milk absorbs the strong garlic flavor. This nourishing soup is particularly good for children. In country districts it was used as a vermifuge.

Soupe de Vie

A simple and inexpensive soup that used to be a great favorite with old people in my part of France—particularly those who were troubled by rheumatism or gout.

Put a quart of water on to boil. When it has reached the boiling point, add a dozen cloves of garlic, a sprig of thyme, a sprig of rosemary and a few bay leaves. I recall that these herbs would always be dropped into the boiling liquid with a symbolic gesture, the way bouquets of flowers might be tossed

into the sea. The soup would then be thickened by the addition
of three tablespoons of olive oil and allowed to simmer for ten
or fifteen minutes. A slice of toasted brown bread would be
placed at the bottom of the soup plate and the hot soup ladled
over that.

Soupe au Farci

The so-called farce is a well-nigh sacred feature in Gascon
cooking. It is used in every dish, with boiled chicken, with
roast pigeon, with stuffed leg of veal. But if you have no
chicken or pigeon or veal with which it can go, well, the farci is
so good in itself that you put it into soup.

Store any bits of leftover bread you may have in an airtight
tin. When you have enough, break up the pieces and soak
them in warm milk. Chop several cloves of garlic, an onion
and parsley. Add a bit of thyme and bay to this. Add some
finely diced bacon or a half-cup of sausage meat. Add two or
three eggs—one per person if you mean to make this your
main dish. Mix all these ingredients thoroughly. In the country
the cook will knead them with her hand so that they are all
pressed together well.

Fry your mixture like an omelette, browning both sides.
When it is well browned and firm, fold it in half, again like an
omelette, and turn it into a sieve, which you then lower into
your boiling soup. Let it simmer for a quarter of an hour. If you
do not have a proper sieve but have some good cabbages growing in your garden, go out and pick one of the large outer leaves.
Drop the cabbage leaf into boiling water in order to soften it,
then wrap your little packet in the cabbage leaf and lower this
gently into the soup. Now you will be able to eat your *farci*,
wrapping and all.

Whatever soup you are having, whether it be beef broth
or vegetable soup, it will be greatly enhanced by the *farci*.

Now when you come to serve your soup, gently lift out the
little packet, which will have puffed out nicely but still have
retained its shape. Bring it to table on a separate plate, to
the great joy of the children who will hurry to finish their

soup in order to be eligible for a big slice of the meltingly soft *farci*, accompanied by some of the vegetables of the soup.

Sour-Milk Soup

This is a great favorite in Poland during hot weather.

Pour a quart of soured milk into a large bowl. Add thinly sliced cucumber, finely chopped sorrel fried in butter, sliced hard-boiled eggs, chopped fennel and a good quantity of finely chopped chives. An ice cube in each plate makes the soup even more refreshing.

You may vary the dish by substituting bits of melon or slices of boiled beets for the cucumbers. The other ingredients remain the same. Thus you have three different soups from one recipe.

Cherry Soup

This dish is highly esteemed in Germany. If you have sour cherries in your garden, do not scorn them. Remove their stems and set the cherries to simmer in a quart of red wine, along with some lemon peel. Add sugar, cinnamon and serve hot with croutons or a slice of toasted bread. Since this soup contains wine, it is not a suitable dish for children.

Queen Margot's Potage

Queen Margot was renowned both for her energy and for her amours. Her favorite soup was made of the leftovers of the chicken she had eaten for dinner. These would be set to cook in milk along with some morsels of bread, a few peeled almonds and a few bay leaves.

After a quarter of an hour's gentle simmering, the bay-leaves are discarded and the rest put through a food mill (or, in our day, a blender). The result is a creamy fragrant soup of virginal whiteness—though virginity was hardly the quality most associated with Queen Margot. But perhaps she had a lingering nostalgia for it. Which may account for this soup.

Sunday Night Soup

For Sunday dinner you may have served a roast chicken, or a duck, pheasant or turkey. Your guests have eaten well and nothing remains of the bird but the carcass. Don't throw it away. It will provide you with your evening meal.

Put the bones and bits of skin in a heavy pot, along with a celery heart diced small, two or three large potatoes and a generous bunch of herbs. Before serving, remove the bones and the herbs. They will have left no trace, except for their flavor.

Chicory Potage

The outer leaves of your head of chicory are too coarse to go into a salad. Save them for a soup.

Cut the leaves into small bits. Fry them in a bit of butter until they are limp. Add a quart of water. Season with salt, pepper and nutmeg. Cover the pot and let it simmer for a quarter of an hour. Then whip in the yolks of two eggs and serve it with croutons or a slice of toasted bread.

"Little Cousin" or Mallow Soup

This is one of the most attractive soups I have ever eaten. The country name for mallows is "little cousins," which explains the name of this dish. Go out into your garden and gather a selection of whatever greens you have growing there —a handful of spinach, a handful of sorrel, some leaves of Swiss chard, the outer leaves of chicory and one or two leeks. Add a large bunch of wild mallow leaves. Chop the various greens up small and set them to boil in a quart of water. Before serving, add a cup of fresh cream or a beaten egg.

You may make a richer soup by adding a knuckle of veal to the pot. This means longer cooking—perhaps an hour or more. But you will have a complete and succulent meal.

Purslane Soup

Purslane is a common garden weed with high nutritive value and a unique taste. Do not hoe the plants up ruthlessly; save a few for cooking. They are spreading plants with thick leaves and reddish stalks.

Pick a cupful of the leaves and wash them carefully, for they tend to be gritty. Drop them into a quart of boiling water or meat stock. Add some lettuce leaves or some sorrel, some green beans or peas, some chervil, a chopped onion and a bit of sugar. Let the mixture simmer for a quarter of an hour. At the end, add a dash of fresh cream or a lump of butter and serve the soup with croutons or toasted bread.

Tarragon Soup

Set a half-pound of dried peas on to boil in a quart of water. When they are almost soft, add a generous handful of fresh tarragon. Put the soup through a food mill and add a bit of butter or fresh cream.

Pea-pod Soup

You have picked a basketful of green peas in the garden. After shelling the peas, do not discard the pods. Set a quart of the pods to boil in an equal quantity of water, along with a bunch of mixed herbs. Put through a sieve to remove the hard shells. Add a lump of butter and serve with croutons.

Nettle Soup

Gathering your nettles is the hardest part of the job. But if you have already weeded out a patch from your garden, do not throw them away. You can make a wonderful and nourishing soup from them.

Cut up a large onion and fry it in a bit of olive oil. Chop the nettles and add them to the pot. Stir with a wooden spoon for about five minutes. Add a quart of water. Let this simmer for a quarter of an hour. Put a spoonful of fresh cream or a nut of butter into each plate and ladle the nettle soup on top. The consistency of this soup is particularly agreeable, for the dangerous nettles turn to sheer velvet.

Radish-top Soup

You have served your family a bunch of freshly picked red radishes for lunch. Do not discard the tops. They can make an excellent soup, extremely rich in iron.

Treat the radish leaves just as you would the nettles in the previous recipe. If your hungry family seems to need a somewhat more substantial dish, you may add a few potatoes, cut small to speed their cooking.

A Meatless Pot-au-Feu

You can make an excellent *pot-au-feu* without using meat. You will use cheese instead.

Select a heavy pot such as you would make stew in. Brown an onion in a bit of olive oil. Add potatoes, carrots and whatever other vegetables you would normally use for *pot-au-feu*. Add a generous bunch of mixed herbs and enough water to cover the vegetables. When the pot is simmering, throw in a large piece of gruyère cheese—say, half a pound. By the time the vegetables have softened, the cheese will have quite disappeared. But the dish will have taken on the taste of meat —you would swear there was meat in it.

This is a highly nourishing dish for vegetarians.

Cold Sorrel Soup

This would be a fine company dish on a hot summer day.

Chop a half-pound of sorrel. Put it to boil in a quart of water for ten minutes. Add salt and pepper and a bit of chili powder.

Pour the soup into a tureen and let it cool. Add the juice of a lemon, two large garlic cloves chopped fine, and sprinkle the surface with cucumber slices, sliced hard-boiled eggs and parsley.

Place the tureen in the refrigerator and chill thoroughly. If you have been caught short on time, you may chill it quickly by adding some ice cubes immediately before serving.

Gazpacho

This dish originated in Spain where the torrid summers call for a really fresh soup.

Fill your tureen with the following: a selection of herbs, cut fine; a handful of finely chopped scallions; a quarter of an onion; a number of cucumbers, finely diced; a slice of crumbled bread, several chopped tomatoes, and half a green pepper. Add a jug of water, some ice cubes, a dash of lemon juice, two or three tablespoons of olive oil, salt and pepper. Sprinkle the surface with oregano.

In Spain, this soup is always served in cups. It makes a fine prelude to an evening meal on a hot summer day.

There are innumerable versions of Gazpacho. If you like a smooth soup, put the mixture through a blender, except for the herbs.

Vegetable Juice

You may wish to start your meal with a glass of vegetable juice. Pack your juicer with the following: one carrot, two or three stalks of celery, one cabbage leaf, one tomato, a cucumber spear, a lettuce leaf, one small onion, some herbs, etc. Whirl and serve in a tall glass, seasoned with a dash of lemon juice, salt and pepper.

Main Dishes

Boiled Chicken, Henry IV Style

"I would like to see every workingman in my kingdom have a chicken in the pot on Sunday," said good King Henri, thus proving that he was genuinely concerned about his subjects' welfare. For though a chicken in the pot is not the be-all and end-all of happiness, it is certainly one of the components of it.

The kind of chicken the good king meant would not have been the fat capon enjoyed by the privileged classes. Your normal boiling fowl is an elderly bird who has laid more than her share of eggs. She is somewhat sinewy but has no lack of flavor. Such a chicken requires long, slow cooking, and is best stewed along with an assortment of vegetables such as carrots, onions, turnips, celery and mixed herbs. To make the dish more festive, the bird may be stuffed with the *farci* whose recipe I have already given. The opening should then be sewed up with heavy thread.

Serve the bird on a large platter surrounded by the vegetables with which it was cooked, the stuffing, a mound of rice and perhaps a tomato sauce.

This is the classic family dish in southwest France and is indispensable at every solemn occasion, whether it be a wedding or some rustic banquet celebrating the harvest or the grape-gathering. At Gavarret my Aunt Marie still serves it whenever we have a family gathering.

Galimfrey

Here is a medieval recipe that deserves to be revived.

You have served a leg of roast mutton for dinner. There is quite a bit left. Trim the meat off the bone, cut it into small pieces and set it to simmer in a glass of grape juice, along with some capers, some raisins, a chopped onion, some chives, a pinch of cinnamon, a few cloves, a bit of bacon or salt pork and a spoonful of sugar. Let the mixture cook gently for about a quarter of an hour.

For a more festive effect you can flambé this dish at table. Pour a glass of warm cognac or armagnac over it and set it alight.

They did some things well in the Middle Ages, didn't they?

Rabbit with Prunes

Prunes make an excellent accompaniment to meats of all sorts. In my part of France we have devised hundreds of ways of using them, each more delicious than the next.

Take a cut-up rabbit and set it to marinate for twenty-four hours in a quart of red wine to which you have added a glass of armagnac, a bunch of mixed herbs, some slices of onion, salt and pepper. Meanwhile, you are also soaking a half-pound of prunes.

Remove the pieces of rabbit from the marinade and brown them in a stew pot with some bits of salt pork. Then add the marinade and let your pot simmer gently for half an hour. Then add the prunes and let it all cook fifteen minutes longer.

A similar dish may be prepared with beef.

Stuffed Poultry with Prunes

All poultry suitable for roasting (chicken, duck, guinea fowl, turkey) will be enhanced by a prune stuffing. Soak about a third of a pound of prunes in water. Slit them and remove the pits. Chop them and add an equal quantity of sausage meat, two diced apples and a third of a cup of dried raisins. Brown the liver of your fowl in butter and add it, chopped, to the above mixture. Stuff the cavity of the fowl with the mixture and sew up the opening.

Another prune stuffing: Soak half a pound of prunes overnight. Remove the pits—they slip out easily when the prunes are completely soft. In place of the pit insert a bit of lean bacon into each prune. Fill the cavity of your bird with these, sew up the cavity and bake.

Chicken with Capon

In my part of France, we like to slice a loaf of bread lengthwise and rub the crust with garlic. This we call "making a capon." A capon is, of course, also the castrated rooster, which grows large, fat and succulent. The following recipe plays on this ambiguity.

Take a good piece of crust from a country bread. Crush several cloves of garlic and rub its outside well. Now slit the breast skin of your roasting chicken and insert the crust under the skin. Your chicken looks much larger and plump-breasted—a mock capon. Place a few cloves of garlic in the cavity of the bird, along with its liver and giblets. Set it to roast. The bread absorbs all the juices and becomes particularly delicious. When the time comes for serving, remove the "capon" and divide it equally among the guests so that no one feels cheated.

You might also garnish your roast chicken with a circlet of toasted crusts that you have rubbed with garlic. If you have some extra livers, brown them in butter, sprinkle them with chopped garlic and douse them with a spoonful of armagnac. Spread these on your crusts. Again, make sure you have enough for each of your guests.

Pot Roast, Polish Style

This is the gala dish in Poland. You must start marinating your meat three days before you mean to cook it.

Take a solid piece of beef, three or four pounds in weight. Rub it with coarse salt and lard it with bits of salt anchovy. Prepare the following marinade: one cup of wine, one cup of water, one cup of vinegar, a handful of baby onions, a spoonful of cloves, several slices of lemon, four or five bay leaves, a handful of basil, several sprigs of thyme and savory, a few juniper berries and a pinch of ground ginger. Bring this mixture to a boil and pour it over your beef. Turn your beef every day for two more days.

Roast your beef in a heavy, covered kettle, basting it frequently with the marinade to which you have added a cup of sour milk. Serve the meat along with a hot sauce composed of the marinade thickened by a few spoonfuls of flour and seasoned with chopped anchovies and capers.

Herb Omelette

I once had lunch at the Lake Como house of one of the great gourmets of Italy, a man deeply versed in the science of herbs and author of several books on that subject. We had some omelettes and I can swear that they were the most delicious I have ever eaten.

Everyone knows the omelette of mixed herbs which contains a medley of chopped herbs like parsley and chervil. But my Italian friend served me with a succession of tiny omelettes, each one containing a different herb. One was of parsley, one was of chives, one of tarragon, one of thyme, one of sage, one of basil, one of mint.

This might be a wonderful idea to try on your friends. Just as you serve an assortment of cheeses, you might serve an assortment of omelettes. You might identify each kind, or let people guess.

Velvet Eggs

A splendid way to eat onions. There are several versions of this recipe but the principle remains the same.

Cut up five or six large onions and fry them in a little butter over gentle heat until they are yellow. Then add half a cup of white wine and let the onions poach a few moments until they are soft. Prepare a classic *béchamel* sauce and add this to the onions. Butter a shallow earthenware dish, or individual ramekins, and cover the bottom with this mixture. Top with hard-boiled eggs cut in half and a dusting of grated cheese. Brown under the broiler for a few minutes.

My Aunt Marie tells me that she adds a speck of sugar and a bit of vinegar to her *béchamel* sauce after the onions have gone in. This makes the dish even tastier.

Onion Tart

This makes an excellent main dish. Cut up two pounds of onions and fry them in butter or olive oil until they are yellow. Prepare a pie crust and line a shallow baking dish with it. Spread your onions evenly over the bottom. Now beat up two eggs and a cup of milk. Add salt and pepper and pour this over your layer of onions. Set it to bake. When the crust is done (about thirty minutes), the tart is ready.

Chicken with Onions

Instead of the usual assortment of vegetables, you will use exclusively onions. Peel as many as you can without tears —you should have at least a dozen. Insert two or three cloves into one of the onions and throw them all in, whole, along with your chicken. Add a bunch of mixed herbs and simmer gently for an hour or so.

The liquid of this dish is particularly tasty, and the onions will have become marvelously soft and melting. Rice makes a good accompaniment to this dish.

Stuffed Breast of Veal

If you have developed a taste for the *farci* I described earlier, you can use it in a host of other dishes. It is a fine stuffing for a breast of veal.

You will want to prepare a large quantity of this stuffing, for there is never too much of it. If you have more than your meat will hold, you can always wrap it in a cabbage leaf and cook it alongside.

Have your butcher prepare the breast of veal for stuffing. Fill the pocket with your stuffing and stitch up the opening with heavy thread.

Treat the breast of veal as you would a pot roast and set it to cook gently in a closed kettle along with as many vegetables as you can find—carrots, turnips, celery, cabbage, leeks, etc.

The dish is as good cold as it is hot and the meat can easily be carved into neat slices.

Carbonade

This is a Flemish recipe but it appeals to me because it uses a generous amount of onions, just as does my native cuisine.

Brown a number of small steaks, either on the grill or in a heavy pan. Chop a good quantity of onions and fry them in lard until they are yellow. (We are cooking Flemish style, which means we use lard instead of olive oil.) Cover the bottom of your heaviest stew pot with a thick layer of these onions. Place your steaks on top of this and cover them with still another layer of onions. Add a bunch of mixed herbs, salt, pepper and a pint of beer. Cover and let the pot simmer over gentle heat for an hour or more until the steaks are soft. Serve with mashed potatoes or rice, and a good bottle of beer.

Gasconnade

A *gasconnade* is a boast, a brag. It is also the name of a delicious dish. Though the recipe is of the simplest, the result is something to brag about.

You have bought a good leg of mutton. Have the butcher remove the bone. (Or you may do it yourself if you are skillful at this sort of thing.) Now fill the place where the bone has been with as many cloves of garlic as it will hold. Sew the incision up with strong thread and set your leg of mutton to bake in the oven.

When you carve the roast, you will be surprised to find almost no trace of the garlic. But its taste will have impregnated the meat through and through.

Roast Pork with Herbs

Blend together a bit of thyme, some crumbled bay leaf, sage, a quarter of a teaspoon of cloves, a sprinkle of pepper, a quarter of a teaspoon of nutmeg and a tablespoon of coarse sea salt.

Rub your pork roast with this mixture. Let it stand for several hours before consigning it to the oven. Baste it every hour with a mixture of one-half water, one-half white wine.

The spices will become encrusted in the crackling and the taste will be delicious.

Marinated Pork Roast

Pork has an affinity for the aromatic herbs which we should take advantage of. Prepare a marinating solution including olive oil, lemon juice or vinegar, chopped garlic, sliced onion, thyme, bay leaf, sage, pepper and sea salt. Soak your pork roast (whether loin, ham, shoulder or butt) in this marinade for two days, turning several times so that the meat is well impregnated with the marinade.

Set to bake, basting it every hour with the marinade.

Salmagundi

The best *salmagundi* is made in Bayonne, because the key ingredient of this dish is Bayonne ham. If you were sensible enough to have bought a Bayonne ham during your vacation trip and have a bit left, use a thick slice of it. If not, ask your butcher for a Bayonne ham bone. There is always a good deal of meat left on a ham bone.

Trim the last of the meat off the bone—even a morsel of it goes a long way. Put the ham at the bottom of a heavy casserole. Fill your casserole with a mixture of onions, green beans, fava beans, green pepper, two or three baby artichokes cut in quarters, a few cloves of garlic and a bunch of mixed herbs. Braise in olive oil for a few minutes. Then add two cups of white wine, cover and let simmer gently for half an hour. Add two or three small heads of lettuce ánd some cherry tomatoes. Simmer for another half-hour. Then bring it to table.

Sauces

Mint Sauce

We do not make nearly enough use of mint in France. However, the English, though they are generally considered uninventive in cuisine, have an excellent mint sauce to their credit. Let us borrow their recipe.

Pick a bunch of fresh mint from your garden or from the bank of a nearby brook. Strip the leaves and cut them fine. Place them in your sauce boat and add four tablespoons of sugar, two tablespoons of wine or cider vinegar, four tablespoons of water, salt and pepper.

Serve this sauce fresh as an accompaniment to lamb, whether hot or cold.

Sage Sauce

Here is another recipe borrowed from the English. (Of course, they are welcome to any of ours in exchange.)

Cut up two large onions and brown them in butter or drippings. Add two slices of bread softened in milk and two large spoonfuls of chopped sage leaves. If you have no fresh sage available, dry sage will do. Pour the juices of your roast on this, whether pork, veal, duck, and serve it from a sauce boat. You may also fill the cavity of your duck with the mixture, and remove it after roasting, to be served in the sauce boat along with the gravy.

Herb Sauce for Fish

Today your menu calls for poached fish. Here is something to dress it up with. Make a *court bouillon* using one sprig of thyme, one sprig of basil, one sprig of savory, one sprig of marjoram, one sprig of sage, two chopped shallots and a handful of chives. Add salt, pepper and a pinch of nutmeg. Let the herbs simmer in the bouillon for ten minutes, then strain.

Thicken the sauce with a *roux* made of one tablespoon of flour and a bit of butter. Let it boil gently for a few minutes. Just before serving, add the juice of a lemon and a pinch of chervil and tarragon. Your plain poached fish will be worthy of a three-star restaurant.

Green Sauce

A way of adding fillip and high vitamin content to ordinary mayonnaise.

Add a small quantity of boiling water to a handful of cress, a handful of spinach leaves, some sprigs of chervil, parsley and tarragon. Cook the greens for five minutes. Then put them through a blender. The result will be a thick green purée. Blend the purée into a bowl of mayonnaise. This is particularly attractive served with cold fish or lobster salad.

Mixed Herb Sauce

Melt two tablespoons of butter in a small frying pan. Add two tablespoons of flour and blend. Add a handful of finely minced herbs: parsley, shallots, chives, tarragon, chervil, perhaps lamb's lettuce and cress. Add a cup of gravy and cook until it thickens, about fifteen minutes. Serve warm with a veal or pork roast.

Poor Man's Sauce

The humblest of the sauces, and the quickest to make. Simmer a bunch of parsley, cut fine, and five or six chopped shallots in a small quantity of water. Add salt, pepper and a tablespoon of vinegar. Let it cook gently for a few minutes. This will dress up the remains of a roast or boiled beef.

Garlic Butter

Mash two or three cloves of garlic and mix with a good lump of butter. A dab of this butter on top of a grilled steak adds a distinctive note.

Currant Sauce

This is a tart sauce often served in Germany with poultry or roasted veal.

Pick a pound of currants from your bushes; they need not be completely ripe. Wash them, strip them from the stalks and cover them with boiling water for a few minutes. Then pour off the water and put the currants in a heavy saucepan along with a cup of wine, some sugar, cinnamon, grated lemon peel, a tablespoon of butter and a dash of salt and pepper. Let the mixture cook gently—the fruits should keep their shape. At the last moment thicken with some bits of bread and serve hot from a sauce boat.

Rosehip Sauce

You can make a similar sauce with ripe rosehips. Blanch the hips in boiling water and rub away the browned stamens and the fluff.

This makes a lovely red sauce with a unique flavor.

Holy Water Sauce

Here is a recipe that goes back to the Middle Ages. It was good enough, so the saying of the time went, to be given to the Lord God Himself without confession. You will want a goblet of rosewater and a goblet of grape juice, a speck of powdered ginger and a pinch of marjoram. Boil all these together for a few minutes, then strain. This sauce goes particularly well with Easter lamb.

Pimpernel Sauce

Put a sprig of pimpernel or oregano into a bowl along with a sprig of tarragon, a sprig of chervil, a sprig of cress and two chopped shallots. Add salt, pepper and a dash of vinegar. Cover with a cup of boiling water. Let the mixture steep for an hour or two, then strain. Thicken the liquid with a spoonful of flour and a bit of butter and serve hot with either meat or fish.

Vegetables

Stuffed Cabbage

This makes a meal in itself and is a fine way to deal with a full-grown cabbage, which is too often considered the poor relation in the garden.

Set some water boiling in a large kettle, along with a dash of salt. Now place your cabbage in the kettle and let it boil for five minutes. Take it out, drain it and carefully separate the leaves one by one, so that it looks like an open flower. Meanwhile prepare the stuffing, which I described in Chapter 3. To be sure, there are other kinds of stuffing, but I am partial to this one, because it contains so many healthful herbs.

When you have stuffed your cabbage bountifully, press the leaves gently together and tie it round with a bit of string. Now set it to cook again, as you would a *pot-au-feu*. You may surround it with all sorts of other vegetables such as carrots, onions and turnips.

Some people prefer to detach the cabbage leaves and wrap each one separately about a portion of stuffing. The packets are then laid carefully into the heavy kettle and stewed slowly. I myself prefer the cabbage to remain whole: a stuffed cabbage is a majestic and comforting sight. It may easily be carved in portions like a cake. But either way, stuffed cabbage is delicious.

Stuffed Cabbage with Chestnuts

If your family has enjoyed your stuffed cabbage, you can surprise them with a variation.

Prepare a purée of fresh chestnuts. This is a rather complicated affair and you may prefer to buy a can of puréed chestnuts. While I do not generally approve of canned foods, in this case I will make an exception. Add half a pound of lean bacon, diced very small, or the same quantity of sausage meat. Season with salt, pepper and a dash of nutmeg.

Stuff your cabbage with this mixture, as in the previous recipe. But instead of cooking it over a slow fire, bake it in the oven, basting it occasionally with a mixture of boiling water and butter.

You may invent all kinds of stuffing for your cabbage. Its fine big leaves will hold whatever you choose to fill them with, and the mingling of flavors is always glorious.

Eggplant Caviar

A favorite recipe in Bulgaria, where it is the caviar of the poor man and the shepherd.

Bake some small eggplants whole over a grill or in the oven. A wood fire makes them particularly tasty. When they are soft, remove them from the fire, let them cool, cut them in half and scrape out the pulp with a spoon. Now crush three or four large cloves of garlic in a mortar and mix with some olive oil, stirring this as you would a mayonnaise. Combine with the eggplant pulp and stir well. Season with salt and pepper.

This may be served either hot or cold. It makes a wonderful spread on toasted bread.

Cabbage with Milk

People who ordinarily turn up their noses at cabbage will find this a delicacy. Blanch your cabbage in boiling water for five minutes. Then drain and set the cabbage cooking very gently in milk. By the time the milk is all absorbed, the cabbage is done. Its texture is particularly soft and melting.

Cabbage with Onions

This is an Italian way of cooking cabbage. Cut it in small pieces. Blanch it for a few moments in boiling water. Slice an equal amount of onions. Braise the onions along with the cabbage. A slice or two of bacon in the pan improves the flavor. Do not let the vegetables cook too long—they should be crisp rather than soft.

Red Cabbage with Apples

The Flemish prefer their cabbage cooked until it is very soft. Cut a red cabbage into largish pieces and place these in a heavy kettle with enough water to cover. Add three or four tart apples, peeled, cored and cut in quarters, a bit of salt pork and a few cloves. Cover and let this simmer two or three hours over low heat.

Before serving, drain the juice and season it with a tablespoon of vinegar, two or three spoons of currant jelly and a bit of starch. Boil this sauce down and once more incorporate the cabbage and apples.

Puréed Onions

If this dish appears rarely, it is only because the lady of the house draws back from the prospect of peeling two pounds of onions. Indeed, that takes courage but the dish is worth it.

So open your kitchen window wide or work at your sink under the cold-water faucet. Peel ten, twelve, or fifteen large onions and slice them up. Set them to boil three quarters of an hour in just enough water to cover. Then put them through a food mill or whirl them in your blender. Add a lump of butter and a bit of flour and return mixture to the stove to cook very gently until the paste thickens. Just before serving, whip in two or three tablespoonfuls of fresh cream.

Both in texture and taste this purée is superb. It goes well with any sort of roast.

Onions in the Embers

It used to be customary in the country to bake potatoes in the embers of the fireplace. Sometimes onions were treated the same way. A modern trick would be to wrap the onions, whole and unpeeled, in aluminum foil. They are done after about an hour and become soft and melting. Peel them and eat them with salt.

Eggplant, Squash or Tomatoes in the Embers

Now that people have rediscovered the pleasure of cooking over a campfire or at a barbecue, we can revive some of the old methods of the farmhouse kitchen. But we will use aluminum foil so we do not have sooty casseroles to clean. Eggplant, squash and tomatoes all lend themselves to this type of baking. Eggplants and tender young squash are best sliced and dipped in olive oil and sprinkled with such herbs as thyme, rosemary and sage before being wrapped in their foil envelopes. Tomatoes may be baked whole and sprinkled with herbs afterwards. These vegetables go especially well with brochettes.

Beans with Savory

The broad bean or fava bean is classically cooked with savory, but you may do the same with ordinary shell beans or fresh lima beans. Cook the beans along with a few sprigs of savory until the beans are soft but not mushy. Drain and keep the liquid for a soup, for it is delightfully fragrant. Then lightly fry the beans in a heavy pan with some bits of pork fat. Serve these beans surrounding a roast.

Hops à la Vinaigrette

The young shoots of hops may be treated just like asparagus. They are tender and juicy. Boil them until they are soft and serve with a *vinaigrette* sauce.

Lettuce au gratin

Perhaps your family is not too enthusiastic about salad. Well, there are other ways of getting them to eat their lettuce.

Go out to the garden and pick a large basket of lettuce—you will need at least one head per person. Wash the heads thoroughly and steam them for about ten minutes. They will cook down considerably—in fact, each head will be about the size of an apple. Drain them and arrange them in a heatproof dish. Top with a good thick *béchamel* sauce, sprinkle with nutmeg and grated cheese. Put the dish under the grill until the sauce is bubbly and lightly browned on top.

Stuffed Lettuce

You may stuff lettuce just as you would cabbage. But since lettuces are much smaller, you will want one head per person. Simmer them in bouillon or bake in a slow oven.

Purslane au gratin

The purslane is starting to overrun the garden. You had better do some weeding. Well, there is also good eating there.

Wash the purslane well and blanch it for a few moments to remove any bitterness. Then set it to boil in salted water. Drain and brown it in a frying pan along with a bit of olive oil, garlic and a chopped anchovy. Add a heel of bread, softened in milk. Now place your purslane in an ovenproof dish, dot with bread crumbs and grated cheese, and brown under the broiler.

Fresh Peas with Mint

Again a recipe we are borrowing from the English. Add a sprig of fresh mint to your young garden peas. Before serving, garnish with chopped chives and a bit of butter.

Beet Greens

Cook beet tops as you would spinach. But you had better remove the stems before cooking, for these tend to be tough.

You may treat young buckwheat stalks the same way, or even shoots of wheat. Wild plants such as mallow, borage, plantain and cow parsnip may all be cooked as greens.

Coconut and Vegetable Pudding

This is an interesting way to treat vegetables. The recipe comes from Africa.

Assemble an assortment of fresh vegetables: carrots, turnips, celery, cabbage, fennel, spinach, squash. Cut them up small.

Cook up a quantity of cornmeal mush. Grate an equal amount of fresh coconut and mix with the cornmeal. Now butter a deep mold and fill it with alternate layers of mush and vegetables, ending with a layer of mush.

Steam this pudding in a double boiler for half an hour. Then unmold and serve it on a platter. It looks very handsome and is easily cut in wedges.

Rhubarb Blossom au gratin

Your rhubarb plant is in flower. Cut the big flower as soon as it appears. Cook it like cauliflower—it has almost the same taste. Try it in a white sauce topped with grated cheese.

Dandelion Salad with Croutons

In Gascony we like to put croutons fried with garlic in all our salads. They are especially good with dandelions or shredded chicory.

Grapefruit Salad Dressing

Whip some grapefruit juice with a bit of cream cheese. Season with salt and pepper and serve with crisp salad vegetables like romaine and endive, sprinkled with finely chopped herbs.

Red Cabbage Salad, Heated

This is a popular dish in Poland.

Cut a red cabbage into thin strips and brown it in bacon fat. Add a cup of water, a dash of vinegar, salt and pepper. Let it simmer slowly in a covered kettle until it is thoroughly soft. Beat in two yolks of eggs and serve hot. It makes a splendid hors d'oeuvre in the wintertime.

Marinated Cucumbers

Another specialty in Poland, where you will find it on every table, rich or poor.

The ideal container for these pickles would be an old barrel which had held white wine. Lacking that, you may make do with an earthenware crock.

Gather enough cucumbers to fill the crock; place them in layers, interspersing them with a layer of chopped fennel, cherry leaves and a bit of crushed coriander. Make up a heavy brine, heat to boiling and pour over the cucumbers, taking care that they are completely submerged. Place the cover on the crock and let it season for two months before eating.

The fragrant brine is much appreciated by the poor people, who like to soak their bread in it.

American Salad Bowl and Dip

Americans are very strong on vitamins and believe in low-calorie eating. They have created a special dish, the "salad bowl," which permits of endless variations. Raw and cooked vegetables, sometimes fruits, cold meats and fish, are all mingled together and serve as a complete and appetizing meal. French drugstores and quick-lunch bars are now offering the same sort of thing.

Another American creation we might borrow is the dip. This is presented in a large bowl surrounded by a display of raw vegetables: carrot sticks, cherry tomatoes, celery sticks, pretty red radishes, raw cauliflower, daintily trimmed scallions. This dip has become a mainstay of the cocktail hour. It is a welcome alternative to more elaborate hors d'oeuvres, and guests can help themselves to as much or as little as they like. Those who do not care for vegetables are provided with a dish of potato chips or some salt cracker with which they can scoop out their share of dip.

The dip itself is made in the following fashion: Cut up a quantity of herbs—parsley, chives, chervil, etc. Grate an onion and crush a few cloves of garlic. Crumble a bit of roquefort cheese. Mix all this into a pound of cottage cheese. Stir until perfectly smooth. Season with salt and pepper, transfer to an attractive bowl and powder with paprika.

Desserts

Clafouti

This used to be the year-round dessert in French country districts. Each month it was made with another fruit. It would be baked in the tile stove—an impressive structure reaching almost to the ceiling. The clafouti could be baked either directly on the embers or else on the top of the stove.

A batter is made of flour, sugar, milk and eggs. Experienced cooks would do this purely by feel, but I had better provide some measurements. Let us say you will need two cups of flour, one cup of sugar, three eggs and two cups of milk.

Fill a large earthenware baking dish with as much fruit as it will hold and cover with the creamy batter. Set to bake. When the batter is firm and golden, the dish is done. Serve cold, straight from the dish, with a dusting of sugar.

Such a *clafouti* may be made with cherries, apricots, peaches, plums, prunes, apples, pears, white grapes, etc. Blemished fruits, which you might not otherwise want to serve, will do fine in a *clafouti*. Be generous with the fruits, for the crust is only an excuse for them.

Candied Carrots

If your children are tired of eating carrots, there is a way of getting around that. Serve carrots as a dessert. This is an old country trick, dear to our grandmothers who knew how to prepare all sorts of treats that cost almost nothing.

First the carrots must be transformed into fruits, with a wave of the wand. Nothing could be simpler. Peel and slice a pound of carrots. Put them in a heavy pot with enough water to cover them and a pound of sugar. Add grated lemon peel. Cover and cook slowly. By the time the carrots are soft, they will have absorbed most of the water. They are also thoroughly candied. Add the juice of two lemons.

You may use these candied carrots in any number of ways. Make a pretty open-faced carrot tart, or a *clafouti*. Use them to line a charlotte mould, include them in a compote of stewed fruits or in a fruit salad. Use them in an upside-down cake or a meringue pie. They will do well as a substitute for apples. And your children will be delighted with them.

Chestnuts with Fennel

In the good old days it was the custom for the children of the family to go chestnut-picking in the autumn. They would pick huge basketfuls. The chestnuts would then be set to cook, whole, in their skins, along with a stalk of fennel.

The boiled chestnuts would be brought to the table and every member of the family would be given a bowl of hot well-sugared milk. Then everyone would peel his chestnuts and drop them into his bowl of milk. The process was a lengthy one but it allowed time for the chestnuts to sop up the milk. They were then eaten with a tablespoon. The children would be admonished to chew the nuts carefully. This made a glorious complete evening meal.

Raisiné

This preserve used to be made on every farm. I remember
it from my childhood. It enjoyed its day of glory during the war,
when sugar became unobtainable. Then, people seemed to stop
making it, perhaps because it reminded them too much of
wartime. What a pity, for it is the healthiest of all preserves.
Instead of refined sugar, it makes use of the natural sugar present
in the juice of the grape.

If you are in the country at the time of the grape harvest,
try your hand at it. First, go to some nearby winery where they
are pressing grapes and buy several quarts of fresh juice, from
red grapes. The sweeter the better, but it should not have
started to ferment. Then go to work. You can enlist the help of
your family and friends, for making *raisiné* is a collective enterprise.

I remember how in my childhood the grape juice would be
poured into a great copper kettle and set to heat over a little
wood fire started in the courtyard. Then everyone would bring
the gleanings of the garden or the orchard: melons that had
"gone by," citron, green tomatoes, carrots, apples, pears, quinces,
blue plums, figs, etc. Poor folk might have more vegetables in
their *raisiné*, while the prosperous would tend to have more
fruits. But either way the *raisiné* was delicious.

All day long we peeled our offerings and added them by de-
grees to the grape juice, which bubbled gently in the cauldron.
We started with the hardest fruits, such as quince and carrots,
and added the soft ones later.

I would be given the job of stirring the cauldron with a long
stout stick, practically a club, which had been carefully peeled.
I would have to hold it with two hands, for the stuff would
have gotten very thick. By the time night came, the *raisiné*
would generally be done. But if we had started a bit late, or
lagged somewhat on the job, then the cauldron had to go on
simmering through the night. We would let the fire go almost
out, banking it with ashes, and we would all sleep lightly, taking
turns to go out and stir the pot.

At my Aunt Laurent's they used to take three days to make
the *raisiné*. To be sure, my aunt's *raisiné* contained an infinitude

of ingredients and she would watch over it like a Vestal, never sleeping all the while that it was making.

When the *raisiné* was done, that is, of a burnished brown color and so thick that it could no longer be stirred, it would be ladled out into all the jars, large and small, we had. A few jars would be put up with chopped nuts and some drops of armagnac, to be used on special occasions, and would be so marked with a label.

By the end of winter the *raisiné* would have become so firm in the jars that it would be cut in cubes and eaten like a candy, as is done with quince paste. Grandmothers used to hand out such treats. What a pity that they no longer do so.

A *Simpler* Raisiné

Lacking fruits and vegetables, and the time to peel them, you can nevertheless make a *raisiné* from pure grape juice.

The juice must be simmered gently on a low fire until it has reduced to one-quarter its original volume. This means many hours of cooking. This *raisiné* is almost as delicious as the grander version.

Cider Jam

Not every part of the country is rich in grapes. However, you can make a good preserve from the juice of either apples or pears.

Pear juice is richer in sugar than apple juice and cooks down to a delicious butter. It is best to reduce it first before adding your other ingredients. Reduce it to two-thirds the original volume, then add ripe, sweet fruits and proceed as for *raisiné*.

Elderberry Jam

In August the elderberry bushes are loaded with fruit that is free for the taking. Make use of this bounty of nature, for elderberries furnish an excellent marmalade with laxative properties. Send your children to gather a basketful of the beautiful purple berries. They will enjoy the task and will be glad to help you with the somewhat tedious task of stripping the berries from their clusters. Be sure to wash the berries carefully, because they tend to be dusty.

Weigh the berries and combine them with sugar, using one and a half pounds of sugar to every pound of berries. Cook in a large kettle over low heat until the jam has the consistency of marmalade.

Other wild berries make delicious preserves. The blueberry is highly prized, but did you know that the red fruit of barberry may also be cooked into a jam? As with elderberry, you will require one and a half pounds of sugar to one pound of fruit.

Carrot Jam

It is a common belief that carrots are good for the complexion. And, in fact, the carotene which gives the vegetable its pleasing color will brighten your cheeks. Spread the following jam on your breakfast bread and you will look rosy and well all winter long: Slice up five pounds of carrots. Set them to cook for five hours in five quarts of milk, with two pounds of sugar. Add a bit of lemon peel to improve the flavor. This jam should be kept in the refrigerator, for it is quite perishable.

Honey Jam

Suppose you are fortunate enough to have bees. Instead of eating the honey plain, you may want to use some of it in jams and preserves. With the addition of fruits, the honey loses none of its virtues and lends itself to a great many variations.

You may use pure honey or half-honey and half-sugar for your preserves. But be careful, for honey burns easily. Do your cooking in a heavy pot over very low heat and stir constantly with a wooden spoon. Keep skimming off the froth. Use the same weight of fruits as you have honey. Or, if you are using half-sugar, half-honey, the same weight of fruits as the honey and sugar combined.

Let the mixture boil down until it is very thick. You may treat all your fruits this way: cherries, strawberries, peaches, apricots, apples, pears, plums.

Acacia Flower Fritters

When the acacia trees come into bloom and spread their perfume through your garden, have one of your children climb a tree and bring down some clusters of the blossoms.

Pick off any faded blossoms and dip the clusters one by one in a light batter. Fry them in your iron skillet and serve them with a dusting of powdered sugar.

You may make similar flower fritters out of orange blossoms, violets, elderberry blossoms and even chrysanthemums. White chrysanthemums are the best for this purpose.

Rose Custard

You like to dress up your table with a bouquet of roses when you are having guests. But you can bring roses to your table in still another guise. Your guests will be enraptured by the taste of this dish as well as by its fragrance.

Pick 100 grams of rose petals from your loveliest red roses. Boil them in a pint of water for ten minutes. Let them steep ten minutes longer and strain. Mix this rosewater with a pint of light cream or a can of evaporated milk, and transfer to the top of a double boiler. Cook at moderate heat, over hot, not boiling, water. Custards must never be allowed to boil or they will be tough and stringy. Add sugar to taste (about two-thirds of a cup) and the yolks of six eggs, beaten thoroughly beforehand. Return to the stove and cook, again over hot water, until the mixture begins to thicken. Then remove from heat and allow to cool slightly before spooning into stemmed glass dishes. The glass will allow the delicate rose color of the custard to show to full advantage. Serve very cold, with, perhaps, rose-flavored cookies.

Orange Blossom Custard

Here is another creamy dessert. Scald a quart of milk. Add two-thirds of a cup of sugar and the yolks of six eggs, well beaten. Also add the whites of two eggs. Cook over hot water as described in the previous recipe. Flavor with three teaspoons of orange blossom water. Serve cold.

Violet Paste

Dissolve two pounds of sugar in a pound of apple jelly. Set this to cook over low heat in a heavy kettle. Add a pound of violet petals. Let mixture simmer for ten minutes, no more; violets are fragile.

Jasmine Paste

Jasmine flowers may be treated in the same way as the violets in the previous recipe. Like them, these flowers are fragile and very fragrant. The apple jelly serves as a base and solidifies as the mixture cools.

Candied Orange Blossoms

If you have a grandmother with some experience in candy-making (who, moreover, owns a candy thermometer), ask her to help you with this. If you have no such grandmother, be bold and try it alone.

Collect a pound of orange blossoms. Blanch them in boiling water and drain. Prepare a heavy sugar syrup, boiling it until the mixture "spins a thread." At this point drop your orange blossoms, a spoonful at a time, into the syrup and let the whole thing boil a few minutes longer, for the syrup will have become somewhat diluted by the wet flowers. When it once more "spins a thread," remove the pot from the heat and let the syrup cool. When it is cool enough to touch, lift out the blossoms one by one (each one will be encased in a transparent shell) and spread them out to dry on a sheet of wax paper.

A box of these makes an appropriate gift for a bride and will serve as a charming addition to a wedding feast.

Beverages

Gentian Wine

Why buy commercial *apéritifs* when you can concoct your own, at a fraction of the cost and with a personal touch besides?

Collect a handful of gentian roots, wash them well and set them to steep in a cup of brandy. If you have a small earthenware crock, that is best for the purpose. After a day add a quart of white wine and let the mixture steep for a week. Serve a small glass of this to your friends on Sunday. Those who are troubled by gout or an incipient flu will be especially grateful.

Marjoram Milk

Scald a pint of milk. Add a few spoons of sugar and two leaves of marjoram, no more. Drink this warm—it is pure nectar.

Eggnog

You are coming down with a cold and have no appetite. Beat up the yolk of one egg in a cup and add warm milk, stirring constantly. Sweeten with honey. This is both food and the best of medicines.

Mulled Wine

More first aid for when you are coming down with a cold. Heat a pint of red wine, preferably in a clay pot. Add two or three spoons of brown sugar, a dash of cinnamon, a few cloves and a bit of lemon peel. Bring almost to a boil. A few slices of lemon in your glass makes this even better. Then betake yourself to your bed under a warm quilt or country eiderdown. You will sweat profusely and wake the next day in tiptop shape.

Rose Honey

This is an old country recipe as poetic as it is delicious.

Your red roses are almost at their end. Hurry and gather their petals while they are still fresh. You will need about 100 grams of rose petals. Put them in a pint of boiling water, boil them for ten minutes, then let them steep for ten minutes longer. Strain through a sieve and add about a pound and a half of honey. Stir well and pour into jars or little crocks.

This keeps excellently. You may use it to sweeten your tisanes or to make pleasant gargles to keep off sore throats in the winter. Thus your roses keep you company all year round.

Blueberry Syrup

Your children have been off by themselves all day gorging themselves on blueberries. They come back with teeth stained blue and a little present for you—at least a quart of the berries, somewhat crushed, to be sure, from being carried in a sheet of newspaper, a large leaf, or someone's lunchbox.

Don't throw the berries away, even if they are the worse for wear. Put them in a saucepan with an equal weight of sugar and simmer them over low heat. Let boil up once or twice, then remove from stove and strain through a sieve. Cool and pour into bottles.

You can make all sorts of delicious syrups out of currants, blackberries, raspberries.

Orange Blossom Ratafia

The orange trees are in flower. Young wives slip a sprig of orange blossom in their hair, for the orange blossom symbolizes happiness. Well, you are no longer so young, so you put your happiness into bottles.

Steep 50 grams of orange blossom in a quart of brandy for four days. Strain and add half a pound of sugar dissolved in a pint of water. Then bottle this. On opening your bottle, the perfume of orange blossom will pervade the room. This makes a calming after-dinner liqueur, and prepares you for pleasant dreams.

Rose Ratafia

Gather rose petals. The color matters less than the fragrance. You will want about 150 grams of petals. Steep them in a pint of warm water for two days. Strain them through a cloth. Mix with an equal quantity of brandy. Add about half a pound of sugar, a dash of cinnamon and a few coriander seeds. Strain once more, after about two weeks, for this *ratafia* should be as clear as crystal. Serve it in your best crystal decanter.

Hippocras

A favorite drink of King Louis XIV.

Add a half-pound of sugar to a quart of red wine. Spike this with a few slices of hot pepper, some ginger, a sliced apple, twelve crushed almonds, twelve cloves and some cinnamon. Let this steep a day and strain it through a sieve. It is perhaps a bit strong on the spices, but after a few glasses of it, you will see as many suns as the Sun King.

A bit of ambergris also went into the original mixture. If you have some, try it, but be careful, for with this addition the drink becomes a powerful aphrodisiac!

Ambrosia

We all know what the gods drank on Olympus. Mix a quart of water with a jar of your best honey. Bring this to a boil and cook until it has reduced to half the original volume. Then add a good glass, or more, of brandy. Bottle this and let it age for ten years or so. Of course, you may sample some from time to time.

Bachelor's Liqueur

You can put up some of your garden fruits in brandy. The best for this purpose are cherries, plums, currants, grapes and blue prunes. There are a few exceptions—strawberries and raspberries, because they are too fragile. Apricots and apples, too, do not lend themselves well to this treatment.

However, here is a method for brandying every fruit imaginable in a wonderful rich mixture of tastes and textures. You will want a large crock, holding at least a gallon. Start with a pint of pure grain alcohol and warm it slightly. Then as the months go by, add whatever ripe fruit you have. You will probably start with cherries, then strawberries, raspberries, apricots, peaches, prunes, pears, grapes. Oranges, too, can go into it. You will want to pit the fruits, except for the cherries. Sprinkle each layer of fruit with sugar. In October, add a pint of old apple brandy. Seal the crock and put it on a high shelf.

Open it at Christmas and dole it out to your friends.

9. A Way of Life After My Heart

Not long ago a critic said of my doctrines: "Mességué would have us go back to the age of food-gathering." To be sure, he meant to ridicule me and expose me as a reactionary. Still, it was a telling phrase my critic coined and one I do not altogether reject. For I am a gatherer, both literally and figuratively. This is my primary attitude toward life and I can only be grateful to the critic who defined it so aptly. "Gather life's roses," we are advised by Ronsard, the prince of poets. And I, too, keep insisting that we must all leave room in our lives for gathering. We must gather not only roses but field flowers and wild herbs and fruits and berries, and we must stoop our backs to gather them and strain upward for branches just beyond our reach and make great bouquets of our pickings and fill our baskets to the brim and breathe in the scents and fragrances of our booty and eat of what we have found with gusto.

This is how I look upon gathering, which I consider both the noblest and the most natural of human sports—and, in this era of increasing leisure, a sport that should be rediscovered. Gathering is no longer an easy matter, I must admit. Most of us cannot step outside our doors and find nourishment in the nearest hedgerow. Nature has made herself a bit scarce and unattainable, perhaps because she is proud and wants to prove that she is not so easily conquered as man in the last century has tended to assume. But she is still there and will bestow her favors on those who seek her out respectfully.

So on your weekends and vacation trips seek out nature and pay her proper homage. Bring back some of the treasures of the fields: bunches of wild thyme, lavender, mint; a garland of garlic and a sack of onions; some farm-cured ham and sausages; a jar of honey.

Keep up relations throughout the year with your country acquaintances. They will be glad to send you some of their produce and gratified that you prize it. Quite a few people have asked me to put them in touch with farmers in my neighborhood who are willing to sell good country fare, and I can vouch that the resultant transactions have been satisfactory to both sides. In fact, a number of friendships have been born this way. Not only have parcels been sent, but postcards have been exchanged and children have visited back and forth during vacations.

On the basis of such parcels, a number of my friends have formed such happy associations with the Gers, with which they previously had no ties, that they have ended by buying houses there, intending to use them first for vacations and eventually for retirement. One of them has even sold his villa on the Riviera in order to acquire property close to Fleurance. To be sure, in his case there was a prior history of a connection with my native village of Gavarret. And not only with my village, but—to bring the story very close to me—with my own aunt, Marie Laurent. But let me tell how all this happened.

My aunt, Marie Laurent, is a rather exceptional person and has been so recognized by her neighbors, who have elected her mayoress of the town. I have always called her Godmother because she carried me to the baptismal font, but I am only one among many for whom she has been godmother over the years. In some ways she resembles those fairy godmothers who turn pumpkins into coaches and rags into finery. In other ways she resembles those good ladies of wartime who adopt a number of soldiers and send them parcels of homemade goodies to improve their morale. My aunt's parcels, I guarantee, are tremendous morale raisers.

I often go to see her in her big house surrounded by flowers on the outskirts of Gavarret. My father was born in this house and it has belonged to the Mességué family for five centuries. My aunt has appointed herself custodian of the family archives and has shown me records dating from 1600 which she has found in the attic. But if I enjoy visiting her, it is not solely to discuss family history. It is rather the present atmosphere of the house that draws me. When I come unannounced, as I sometimes do,

I find my aunt busy at tasks that fill the whole place with delightful perfumes. What my aunt can accomplish in a single day is positively staggering. Not only does she direct all the farm work, but she also manages to put up literally hundreds of jars, bottles and crocks of good things from the farm, which she then sends out to her various protégés all over the country.

Sometimes I bring her the address of a client of mine. "Here's somebody else, Godmother, who would be so pleased if he could place orders with you. He's a client of mine of long standing."

"That's all very well, my dear Maurice, but my pigs don't yield enough hams for all my customers and my rabbits don't multiply fast enough. I put up hundreds of jars of preserves but my own cupboards are empty. After all, I can't feed the whole world. It's dreadful what people expect."

And to show me how unreasonable people are, my aunt produces the latest batch of mail: "Could you please send me another ham for Christmas? We have almost finished your last one." "We would like to order so and so many sausages, so many jars of preserved goose, so and so many bottles of your aged armagnac." Auntie pretends to be displeased. "That's how it is every day," she grumbles. "There's a limit to what the farm can produce."

During the winter months Aunt will send roasting chickens, guinea hens and fresh eggs to some of her nearby customers. She stops when the weather gets warm, for fear the things will spoil. "What do you think, Maurice," she tells me one day with evident satifaction. "Madame So and So, who buys a chicken from me every week during the winter, never serves chicken during the summer because she can't find any that meet her standards. I can well believe that, too."

It seems to me that both my aunt and her customers benefit from this trade. It could well be imitated on a larger scale. City folk could arrive at similar arrangements with farmers during their vacations, and farmers could take on a number of such customers without its interfering with their regular activities. The extra income is welcome at the farm and the good country things are welcome in the city. A parcel, after all, is always an event, and the more so when every member of the family can enjoy its contents.

"You are not very realistic, Monsieur Mességué," people sometimes tell me. "To depend on parcel post for your fresh eggs and country vegetables is hardly practical, on a large scale."

Yes, of course, I am well aware that such parcels are not the answer to each family's everyday needs. For one thing, the post office could hardly stand the strain. I am not suggesting that a system of food parcels could take the place of regular distribution channels. But the parcels could serve as a supplement. Their real purpose would be to weave threads between city people and country people, from which threads eventually a fabric of understanding and exchange would grow. This fabric could become nationwide and connect up with other such networks elsewhere in the world. For there is no reason why such a system could not be developed anywhere the earth is fruitful.

So seek out the country whenever you can and spend your vacations in peaceful agrarian surroundings. Is it not a blessing to be away from the pressures of the city, the rush of traffic, the polluted air, the endless things to buy, the fatigue and the deadening of the senses? Is it not a high privilege to possess, not the key to the city, but the key to the fields? To be sure, mankind has been expelled from the real paradise, but we can find its nearest equivalent in the country.

I would like to see the city man touch earth and, like the mythic giant Antheus, draw new strength from the contact. For I believe that there is a current of force between the soil and the man who stands upon it. My family has long practiced a bit of sorcery, so I am somewhat sensitive to these matters. I have felt the pull of the earth even without a divining rod in my hands. I know it is there. To walk barefoot on dew-drenched grass in the early morning is not only a physical but a psychic experience. It may surpass any shock treatment for the man who has lost his vital energy.

There are ways to keep this energy flowing even after you have returned, as you must, to the city. There are the parcels of good food that will keep coming and the treasures you have brought back in the trunk of your car. Every time you take a pinch of those herbs you have dried, you will remember where you picked them. What a miraculous thing memory is, and how it can reside in a few dried leaves and shriveled blossoms.

Let all your senses participate in the festival of nature. Innumerable joys come to us through touch and smell and we should not undervalue these small experiences, which seem so simple yet are fraught with such significance. When I pass among the market stalls in Fleurance, I caress the ripe fruits and the magnificent vegetables the way one caresses the curly head of a child. When I am in my herb house, I handle the dried plants from sheer pleasure, and when I stir them about to air them better, the scent they give off is a piercing delight to me.

Pleasures of this sort are well within everyone's means and we can allow ourselves them without stinting. This is my recipe for happiness. I have no streak of saintliness in me and have never preached self-denial or abstinence or even going on a diet. I have always held that a good *cassoulet* partaken with true friends is far easier to digest than some watery leek soup eaten alone in the kitchen or a cursory sandwich gobbled down in a snack bar. To be sure, the *cassoulet* has been prepared with love from good ingredients, while the soup and the sandwich are usually made with no care whatsoever out of lifeless and harmful stuff. But the chief thing is that we look forward to the *cassoulet* because we know it will be good, and the anticipation prepares our stomachs for the forthcoming cheerful little feast. Enjoyment, here, becomes the health factor.

I used to be friends with the good priest Bonaventure Fabron who lived near Nice and, like me, believed in the virtues of plants. When members of his flock came to consult him about the ills of their bodies as well as of their souls, he would give them some packets of herbs, as well as his famous therapeutic brew, now named "Fabronine" in his honor. But before he sent them away, he would always advise his patients: "And from time to time, allow yourself a little spree."

The little spree the good priest recommended could hardly have been sinful. All he meant was that people should now and then have a festive meal in the bosom of their family. Not only would this give their bodies a slight jolt, which is all to the good, but it would also benefit them psychologically.

Earlier in this book I, too, suggested that husbands and wives arrange such private celebrations from time to time. But every family meal can be conceived in this light. The simplest food, eaten in an atmosphere of good cheer and serenity, becomes a feast. And remember that there is no better seasoning for food than laughter. Cultivate the art of laughter within your family circle. It has more to do with love than you may have imagined.

Cultivate, too, the art of loving. If I could choose a personal motto, it would be: "I love to love." We should love things as well as people. Nor should we be afraid of passion because it may involve a certain amount of pain. When I am out among my roses, I often prick myself on their thorns. But I continue to caress my roses because the drop of blood on my finger is of no consequence compared to the rush of blood to my heart that the roses inspire.

People who can no longer feel such waves of rapture are in a sorry way. Blushing should not be reserved for youth alone. There are old ladies who still blush with pleasure when they are given a rose. Do not scoff at them: they are enviable in their girlishness. We should all have things that make us blush with pleasure. It may be something so very simple: a flower that has opened overnight in our garden, some words spoken by a child, some memory of youth, a task well done. The only things that affect us this way are "natural" ones, for any form of artifice is cold and cannot cause these sudden rushes of feeling.

To avoid all passion, to keep one's face expressionless and one's heart like stone, is to prepare for death. Is that the course we want to follow? Is it not better to prepare ourselves each day for life, and let death take us by surprise one night?

Love's power to renew and transform is well-nigh miraculous. How many cases have we not known where desperately ill people whom all had given up for lost have suddenly recovered because they fell in love? Through love, the plain astonish us by turning beautiful and the old by turning young.

Max Jacob has written: "An old man does not say, 'I love you.' He says, 'Love me.'"

To my mind, this is not how it should be. One should be able to say "I love you" at any age. It is the best way to stay young.

Nowadays we all know that sexual activity is not bound up with procreation. Recent research into this question has established that men and women can engage in normal sex relations up to an advanced age, provided that they do not ever discontinue such relations. Neither the menopause nor the male climacteric need be taken as a warning knell in this respect.

I can corroborate this, for I know a good many old fellows in my part of the country who still heartily enjoy marital relations and will even boast of their virility. They have not developed any complexes on this score, unlike city men who are forever exposed, on the movie screen, on signboards, on book jackets, to the sight of young bodies locked in embrace. No wonder they come to feel that this is an exercise reserved for the young.

A neighbor of mine who is close to a hundred—he is, in fact, ninety-five—has confided to me that he still has a certain taste for the sport. "I don't mind telling you, Your Honor," he has said, "that even at my age I sometimes have good moments. When the feeling comes over me, I call upon the ladies. Not here, in Fleurance, because people would talk, but I go to Toulouse."

Not everyone, of course, still cares to call upon the ladies at the age of ninety-five. Perhaps my old neighbor was exaggerating somewhat. He also went to considerable lengths to keep himself in form and would roll naked in the nettles to improve his circulation. I would not want to prescribe such drastic measures to patients of mine who suffer from varicose veins and low blood pressure. Or from sexual indifference. Such advice would be laughed at. Nevertheless, the treatment was obviously good for my old neighbor, who enjoyed excellent health and still had his "good moments."

All through life we should treat sexuality with the respect it deserves. We should not be prudish about it, for it is an essential human function intimately bound up with our entire well-being. Neither should we regard it frivolously, for we thereby cheapen it and reduce sexual union to a mere animal act. This it definitely is not, and we do ourselves a grave disservice by thinking so.

I always hesitate to offer any definite advice on the frequency of sexual relations, though many people ask me for such counsel.

Each individual should follow his own rhythm, according to his age and his state of health. We should also try to achieve a balance in this realm, just as we do in our eating patterns, and avoid both dearth and excess.

To be sure, love is not always to be had, and those cut off from it for one reason or another are to be pitied. But such states should be regarded as mere interludes. We should never deliberately condemn ourselves to emotional solitude, for love will come our way if we are truly searching for it. Those who are inclined to self-abuse should try to avoid sensual stimulation. But if grief has seemed to destroy our whole capacity for physical enjoyment, we should be patient. Sometimes some little thing will prove restorative—embracing a child or stroking a beloved cat or dog. That may be enough to unknot our feelings, and suddenly we realize we are ready for loving again—whatever our age may be.

Sometimes the spirit of love deserts a couple and they enter into a period of coldness. Yet they have only to relearn the simple little gestures of their earlier years—the kindly touches, the tender words they used to exchange, to find themselves once more precious to each other and set out on a second honeymoon—and this can happen at any age.

It seems to me that we can never pay too much honor to the little things that make up love.

Apart from human love, the love of things also sustains our general vitality. I know old men who have remained remarkably youthful thanks to their hobbies. They are deeply devoted to their stamp collection or their vegetable garden, to their old books or their game of *belote*. And this passion is enough to make their blood tingle every day, as sap stirs in the leaves on an old tree in the spring.

Every form of rapture is life-giving. Doctors and psychiatrists have made studies of this matter. Thus it has been found that singing will produce a form of sexual ecstasy in celibate women similar to that of intercourse and that this normalizes the functioning of their hormones. Girls who sing in choruses also experience this happy effect, and perhaps music-making in general offers some such release to the participants. This may explain the quality of joyous calm we find in many musicians.

Alexis Carrel in *Man the Unknown* has stressed the therapeutic aspects of prayer. The effort of the sick to direct themselves toward God, the outpouring of faith and love prayer involves, has such a beneficial effect on certain forms of disease that cures take place, as it were, miraculously. The miracles of Lourdes may possibly be viewed in terms of such sublimation of the body, which raises itself above its sickness. In presenting such an explanation as a serious scientific theory, Carrel became the target of a great deal of criticism. But in recent years science has been moving in this direction and is prepared to acknowledge many facts it previously scorned. Thus this passage from Alexis Carrel may be seen as having a certain prophetic cast:

> The single indispensable element [in the phenomenon of miraculous cure] is prayer. But it is not necessary for the sick person himself to pray, or even for him to possess religious faith. All that is needed is for someone close to him to be in a state of prayer. Such facts are highly significant. They point to the reality of certain relationships between psychological and organic processes—relationships still highly obscure to us but nonetheless actual. They are evidence of the objective importance of spiritual activities which have been ignored by doctors, educators and sociologists. Facts of this sort open up a whole new world.

So if you have religious faith, add a bit of God to all your doings—what sort of God doesn't particularly matter. All forms of God have equal merit, for it is your faith that counts. A bit of God can also enter into your plant-gathering and your soup-making. How much I cannot tell you, this is an ingredient difficult to measure in grams or pinches—perhaps better in puffs or breaths. Well, add a breath of God each time and I am sure you will notice a difference in your results.

There are a number of other elements that go into the composition of the way of life after my heart. I will try to define them, not so that you can imitate me in these things, but so that you can design your own manner of life according to your own tastes and necessities. I myself have a simple standard for telling the good from the bad. I always ask myself: Is this raising or lowering my vitality? And then I know whether what I am doing is right or wrong for me.

What do I mean by vitality? According to the dictionary, vitality is animate existence, vigor, liveliness. In fact, it is the mysterious life force which keeps us going. It is the very pulse and throb of energy in us. Anything that strengthens it is good. Anything that dulls and depresses our vitality is harmful.

Where plants are concerned, we have some sort of yardstick for determining their vitality. We rate them by their germination, their resistance to parasites and extremes of climate (cold, heat), their productivity, their toughness. These qualities are fairly easy to measure.

Where animals are concerned, the terms are somewhat different but the principles remain the same: fertility, resistence to disease, adaptability to climate, longevity, productivity.

Anyone at home in nature—and I wish that we all were—has no trouble recognizing the vitality of a flower or a vegetable. Anyone who has ever thumped a well-grown cabbage or watched over the swelling bud of a rose knows what I mean.

Animals stand even closer to us on the ladder of life and we can even more accurately judge their vitality and marvel at the strength of life in them. Birds, so frail in appearance, exposed to all kinds of weather, can withstand extremes of cold. The rain glides off their feathers, and under the light down that covers their tiny bodies what hot blood courses through their veins.

From what source do animals draw their vitality? From the food they eat, of course. Chickens, for example, think of nothing but eating and will never refuse either grain or worms—which may account for their remarkable fecundity. But animals participate in all the forces of nature. From earliest springtime they warm themselves in the rays of the sun, and this gentle warmth endows them with fresh force. Spring is the season when flowers crop up from the earth and nests are filled with eggs. This blossoming of nature is due to a phenomenon called photostimulation. But how does civilized man respond to this season? Oblivious to spring pressing against our windows, we remain locked up in our houses, our offices and our factories, and when the working day is done, we sit before our television sets.

When a patient appears in my consulting room, I can at once judge his vitality. My method is hardly scientific and perhaps could not be followed by others. But it has served me well. My impressions are almost immediate and I note down on the patient's card "good vitality" or "poor vitality." In the first case, I have observed a sparkle in the eye, a warmth in the voice, a certain pride in the bearing, which are all unmistakable signs of vital force. In the second, I have observed that the eyes are dull, the hair is dry, the skin is gray, the breathing irregular, the handclasp weak and the shoulders bowed—and all these signs have nothing to do with age. There are young people who are already aged and old people who are youthful. Pablo Picasso at ninety was an example of eternal youth.

"It takes a long time to become young," he would say. And he put this belief into practice. He continued to live as a young man lives, expending his force rather than husbanding it, and by so doing he built up an enormous charge of vitality.

We should seize every chance nature puts in our way to recharge our vital forces. A passing ray of sunshine? Quick, run outdoors, lift your face to the light. It will do you good. A heavy shower? Too bad, but go out anyway and let the rain beat against your face; rainwater is wonderful for the skin. Moreover, the falling raindrops have a calming power; they wash away anxiety and relax our nerves.

In the summer expose yourself to the sun, with as little on as propriety permits, and with nothing on whenever you possibly can. The sun's caresses, though they can be searing, are always good for you in moderate amounts.

When winter comes, welcome the cold and harden yourself to it. Go for long walks and breathe in the icy air—the feeling is intoxicating. And do not dress too heavily, but let your body make an effort to counter the cold. When I was young children always went about with bare legs, whatever the temperature. Their knees might be purple now and then, but on the whole they caught cold far less often than the little incubator chicks we raise nowadays.

Similarly, when I was young we could never resist the pleasure of plunging into icy streams. Of course, we would be all shivers afterwards, despite the energetic rubdowns of our friends. After all, we youngsters never had the chance to loll about on Riviera beaches, and swimming pools were very rare in those days.

Automobiles were also rare in our part of the country and youngsters had to use their legs to go to see their friends. This sometimes involved traveling considerable distances and we built up sturdy muscles through walking or bicycling. I am disturbed nowadays at the laziness boys show about any form of physical effort. When I attend sports events, I notice that it is not always the younger members of a team who take part energetically. Quite often you will see fathers of families mount their bicycles for some race, while the younger fellows stand by as careless spectators. I myself take part in any rugby match whenever I have the chance. I used to be a pretty strong player in my younger days and my enthusiasm for the game has not died. My sons also love the game. I always encouraged them to build up endurance, and they will be grateful for this, I hope.

Therefore, if I were to offer some practical advice on how to remain youthful and happy well into one's later years, I would say this: Take nature for your bride. Sleep in nature's bed, even though it be lined with nettles as well as with rose petals. Follow nature's bidding as though she were a beloved wife, and do not play her false. Learn to live at her pace and follow the rhythm of her seasons. Keep close watch of her every moment. Take walks along the back roads to look for the birds in the bushes and the wildflowers in the fields. Pick an apple from a tree and chew it slowly. Drink the newly-pressed wine, also slowly. And pause every so often, in the course of your busier days, to remember the birds, the flowers, the apple and the wine, for these are serene thoughts which soothe your heart and improve your complexion.

Pay court to yourself and treat yourself as well as you can. Montaigne, whose disciple I am in so many respects, used to practice this gentle egotism. To treat oneself well does not mean being indifferent to others. On the contrary, since doing good to others is still another way of causing oneself pleasure, Montaigne's motto was: "Do what pleases you." That, too, is my philosophy.

When as mayor I have a marriage to perform, I always enjoin the couple, in addition to the regular ceremony: "And practice charity toward each other, for that is the highest of the virtues."

I, too, attempt to follow this principle. It is not always easy for me. As I have said before, I am not a saint. Like most Gascons, I have a passionate nature and am often shaken by hatred or anger. But I have to remind myself not to give way to such emotions. Montaigne, I remind myself, would not have approved. To yield to temper is to do harm to oneself. In fact, I have observed that I always feel better for pardoning, forgiving, overlooking vexations. Charity, then, is a sort of balm, a healing lotion that soothes the inflamed feelings. I have set it down on my list of medications, along with rosewater and linden baths.

La Rochefoucauld in his *Maxims* proposed that all our diseases are caused by evil passions. That is, of course, a moralistic point of view with which we are no longer in sympathy. But there is a degree of logic to it. According to La Rochefoucauld, in the Golden Age virtue ruled the earth and mankind knew only happiness. Then came the Age of Iron when the passions were born and evil entered close behind:

> Ambition produced burning fevers and frenzies. Envy begat jaundice and insomnia. From sloth came all the lethargies, paralyses and torpors. Anger caused suffocation, heated blood, and inflammations of the lungs. Fear engendered heart seizures and syncopes. From vanity was madness born. Avarice brought forth scrofula. Melancholy gave rise to scurvy. Cruelty fashioned stones in the bladder and kidney. From slander and false reports came scarlet fever, smallpox and measles, while jealousy bred gangrene, pestilence and rabies.

Two centuries have passed since La Rochefoucauld drew up this inventory of man's afflictions and blamed them on man's deadly sins. To twentieth-century minds, his thesis is of course fantastic. Yet a writer whom we would place in the vanguard of contemporary thought, Alvin Toffler, author of the important book *Future Shock*, has posited a similar line of causation. According to him, our environment is now super-charged with new elements, products of our galloping technology, and as a result of this man is in a state of permanent trauma. This trauma produces an excess of adrenalin in the blood, which manifests itself in the form of anxiety, palpitations and migraine. Thus the headlong pace of progress engenders diseases.

From my own observation of the effect of modern life on the average man I would agree with this. Many of the health problems that come to my attention are traceable, not so much to flaws in the individual's organism, as to the insupportable pressures of modern life. The chemicals in our food are only one example of this. That is why I repeatedly advise a return to older patterns, as well as a sane approach to eating.

Yet we must move forward. I do not contest that. But let the motion be gradual and conscious. Let us set ourselves a firm direction and a reasonable pace, with occasional pauses for rest, self-examination and assimilation of experience. The principal thing is that our lives be dictated, not by driving forces from the outside, but by the interior tempo of our own natures, a rhythm each individual must set for himself.

I have been credited with working magic, but I know no magic charms or spells. All my arts are simple matters of common sense. They are mostly things mankind has always known and always held to. We should not part with these things, for like pieces of furniture long in the family, they stand guard over the happiness of their owners.

Index

Acacia flower fritters, 225
Acupuncture, 137
Adaptive radiation, theory of, 7
Additives
  in animal feed, 11, 182, 183
  in dairy products, 187–88
  in meats, 21–22, 161, 182
  in wines, 11–12
Age and sexual activity, 235–36
Aïgo bouïdo, 196–97
Allergies, 140–42, 163, 164
Almond oil, 165, 166
Ambergris, 146
Ambrosia, 229
American salad bowl and dip,
  219–20
Anemia
  radishes for, 61
  spinach for, 58
  strawberries for, 65
  watercress for, 52
Anesthetics, mint as, 99–100
Angina pectoris
  hawthorn for, 116
  rheumatism and, 134
Animal feed, estrogen in, 11
Animals and herbs, 83, 101, 103,
  105, 106, 108
Antiseptics, 138
  bay leaf as, 93
  mint as, 98
  sage as, 90, 91
  for skin, 158
  in thyme, 86
Aphrodisiacs, 146–48
  celery as, 51
  garlic as, 39–40
  mint as, 99
  nasturtium as, 114
  onions as, 43

perfumes as, 176
savory as, 92
wine as, 191
Apples, 68–70, 126, 173
  red cabbage with, 215
Apricots, 70, 126, 153
Armagnac, 191–92
Arteriosclerosis, 151
Arthritis, 134, 135
  cabbage for, 48
  currants for, 67
  radishes for, 61
  strawberries for, 65
  thyme for, 87
Artichokes, 56–57, 126
Asparagus, 63
Asthma, horseradish for, 61
Astringents
  pimpernel as, 104
  roses as, 112
  yarrow as, 117
Aumont, Marcel, 181

Bachelor's liqueur, 229
Baldness, 175
  nasturtium for, 115, 175
Balsamic moment, 80
Balzac, Honoré de, 147
Bananas, 126
Barley, 186
Basil, 94–95
Baudelaire, Charles Pierre, 154
Bay leaf, 93–94
Baylet, Mme., 28
Beans with savory, 216–17
Beauty, 154–76
Beef
  carbonade, 208
  pot roast, Polish style, 206
Bee stings and rheumatism, 137

Beets, 34, 171
  greens, 218
Berry bushes, 35
Beverages, 190–93
  recipes for, 226–29
Bittersweet (plant), 168
Blackberries, 67–68, 164
Blackheads, 169–70
Bladder, 131–34
Bladder stones
  celandine for, 104
  corn silk for, 118
Bleeding, yarrow for, 117
Blood. See Circulatory system
Blueberries, 68, 172
  syrup, 228
Boileau-Despreaux, François
    Adrien, 139
Boils, 163
Borage, 116, 133
Brambles, 156
Bread, 184–86
  chicken with capon, 205–6
Brillat-Savarin, Anthelme, 146, 177
Bromides in strawberries, 65
Buckwheat, 186
Burdock, 164, 168, 174

Cabbage, 46–49, 125, 135, 136, 163,
    171
  with milk, 215
  with onions, 215
  red, with apples, 215
  red, salad, heated, 219
  stuffed, 213–14
  stuffed with chestnuts, 214
Camomile, 80, 125, 128, 129, 165,
    172
Cancer, 121–22
Candied carrots, 221
Candied orange blossoms, 226
Caoulet, 78
Capon (bread), chicken with,
    205–6
Carbonade, 208
Cardiovascular diseases
  onions and, 44
  rye and, 186
Carrel, Alexis, 238
Carrots, 34, 35, 49–51, 126, 130,
    171
  candied, 221

jam, 224
Castel, Jean-Jacques, 26–28
Celandine, 82, 102–4, 156, 165, 169,
    170, 172
Celery, 34, 51–52
Cellulite, 159–62
  cucumbers for, 55
  ivy for, 108–9
  parsley and chervil for, 84
Cereals, 184–86
Charlemagne (king, France),
    85–86
Cheese, 188
  meatless pot-au-feu, 202
Cherries, 70
  soup, 199
Chervil, 34–35, 84–85
Chest colds, turnips for, 64
Chestnuts
  cabbage stuffed with, 214
  with fennel, 221
Chicken, 179–80, 183
  boiled, Henri IV style, 203–4
  with capon, 205–6
  with onions, 207–8
  Queen Margot's potage, 199
  see also Poultry
Chicory, 58–59, 168, 169
  potage, 200
Children's diseases
  diarrhea, carrots for, 49, 130
  intestinal worms, 41, 44
  nervous disposition, basil for,
    94–95
  radishes for, 61
  teething, mallow for, 109
  of urinary tract, 132
Children's nutrition, 178–79
  carrots in, 49–50
  honey in, 189
  milk in, 187
Chives, 45
Cider jam, 223
Circulatory system, 149–53
  blood in, 152–53
  nettles for, 102
  shepherd's purse for, 111
  watercress for, 52
Cirrhosis of the liver, 190
  cabbage for, 49
Citrus fruits, 126
Clafouti, 220–21

Cleopatra, 165
Coconut and vegetable pudding, 218
Coffee, 145–46, 166, 192
Coffee beans, 42, 44
Colds, 138–40
  chest, turnips for, 64
  currants for, 67
Cold sorrel soup, 202–3
Cologne, 171, 176
Colon bacillus infection, 131
Comfrey, 165
Complexion
  onions for, 44
  see also Face; Skin
Confucius, 121
Conjunctivitis, 172
  celandine for, 103
  parsley for, 85
Cook, James, 47
Copper bracelets for rheumatism,
  137
Cornflowers, 172
Cornmeal, 186
Corn silk, 117–18, 133, 160
Couch grass, 106–7, 133, 158, 160
Cow-parsnip, 117
Creamed garlic soup, 197
Creamed onion soup, 197
Cruciferous plants, 82
Cucumbers, 55–56, 125, 171
  marinated, 219
Cucurbitaceous plants, 82
Curnonsky, 147
Currants, 66–67
  sauce, 212
Custards
  orange blossom, 225
  rose, 225
Cystitis, corn silk for, 118

Dairy products, 186–88
Daisies, 165
Dandelions, 35, 59–60, 126, 133,
  160, 170
  salad with croutons, 218
Decoctions, 123–24
Depuratives
  artichokes as, 56
  celery as, 51
  cherries as, 70
  chicory as, 59
  couch grass as, 107

for face, 168
for furunculosis, 163
nettles as, 102
strawberries as, 65, 66
watercress as, 52
Descamps, Michel, 6–7, 42–43
Desserts, recipes for, 220–26
Diabetes
  asparagus for, 63
  cherries and, 70
  chicory for, 59
  oatmeal for, 186
  strawberries, raspberries and,
    65–66
Diarrhea, 130–31
  blackberries for, 67
  blueberries for, 68
  in children, carrots for, 49
  pimpernel for, 104
  rhubarb for, 65
  roses for, 112
  strawberries for, 66
Digestion
  bay leaf for, 94
  nasturtium for, 115
Digestive, asparagus as, 63
Dips, American salad bowl and,
  219–20
Disinfectant, thyme as, 87, 88
Disintoxicant, grapes as, 72
Disposition, carrots for, 49
Diuretics, 133
  artichokes as, 56
  for cellulite, 160–61
  cherries as, 70
  chicory as, 59
  corn silk as, 118
  couch grass as, 107
  cucumbers as, 55
  currants as, 67
  dandelions as, 60
  garlic as, 42
  nettles as, 102
  onions as, 44
  peaches as, 70
  plums as, 71
  strawberries as, 65, 66
Dizziness
  lavender for, 105
  mint for, 98
  watercress for, 53
Dumas, Alexandre, 36

Dysentery
  blueberries for, 68
  pimpernel for, 104
  roses for, 112

Echnernier, Dr., 149, 150
Eczema, 140, 162–64
Eggnog, 227
Eggplant
  caviar, 214–15
  in the embers, 216
Eggs
  as shampoo, 174
  in skin treatment, 169
  velvet, 207
Elderberry jam, 223–24
Elizabeth (queen, Hungary), 88, 89
Emetic, violets as, 114
Essence of Youth, 70, 156
Estrogen in animal feed, 11
Eyes, 172
  blueberries for, 68, 172
Eyewashes, 172
  celandine as, 103
  dandelion for, 60
  parsley as, 85

Fabron, Bonaventure, 234
Face, 166–71
  see also Skin
Farci
  soupe au, 198–99
  veal stuffed with, 208
Fats, 182
Fennel, 34, 62–63
  chestnuts with, 221
Fertilizers, 8
Fever, borage for, 116
First-aid
  cabbage as, 47–48
  shepherd's purse as, 111
  yarrow as, 117
Fish, 184
  aïgo bouïdo, 197
  herb sauce for, 211
Fleurance, France, 2–3, 16–26, 28, 29
Fleurance (company), 26–28, 30
Flowers, 18–19
Foie gras, 183
Four-flower tea, 109, 139
Foxgloves, 151

France, Ministry of Nature of, 13
Fritters, acacia flower, 225
Fruits, 64–73
  bachelor's liqueur, 229
  clafouti, 220–21
  recipes for, 220–24
  see also names of individual fruits
Fruit trees, 35
Fungicides, 6
Furunculosis, 162–63

Galen, 119
Galimfrey, 204
Gardening, vegetable, 33–39
Garlic, 39–43, 138, 139, 141, 147, 150–51, 153, 164
  butter, 212
  gasconnade, 209
  soup, 196
  soup, creamed, 197
Gasconnade, 209
Gathering herbs, 74–84, 230
Gavarret, France, 1
Gazpacho, 203
Gentian, 153
Gentian wine, 226–27
Geraniums, 35
Gers, France, 19–20, 29–30
Gilles, Louis, 24–25
Gingivitis, roses for, 112
Gonorrhea and rheumatism, 134
Gooseberries, 66–67
Gout, 134
  parsley and chervil for, 84
  rosemary for, 88
  spinach, warning against, 58
  strawberries for, 65, 66
  tomatoes for, 57
Grapefruit salad dressing, 219
Grapes, 71–73, 126, 130, 170
  raisiné, 222–23
Grasse, France, 10
Greens
  beet, 218
  salad, 53–54, 126
Green sauce, 211
Gums. See Teeth, mouth and gums

Hair, 174–75
Ham, salmagundi, 210
Hawthorn, 115–16, 151
Hay fever, 140–41

Headache, mint for, 99
Heart, 149–53
  hawthorn for, 115, 116
Heather, 133
Hederin, 108
Hedge mustard, 139
Hemingway, Ernest, 191–92
Hemlock, 82, 84
Hemorrhages, pimpernel for, 104
Hemorrhoids, 152
  blueberries for, 68
Henri IV (king, France), 39–40,
  147, 179, 191, 203–4
Herbicides, 6–8
Herbs, 74–118
  gathering, 74–84, 230
  omelette, 206–7
  roast pork with, 209
  sauce, mixed, 211–12
  sauce for fish, 211
  see also names of individual herbs
Herpes, 163
Hiccups, tarragon for, 95
Hippocras, 229
Hippocrates, 36, 52, 122
Hollyhock, 109–10
Holy water sauce, 213
Honey, 164, 188–89
  jam, 224
  rose, 227–28
Hops, 148–49
  à la vinaigrette, 217
Horse chestnuts, 152
Horseradish, 60–62, 173
Horsetails, 152
Hypertension, 150

Impotence, 145
Infusions, 123, 124
Insect bites
  currants for, 67
  parsley for, 85, 165
  rheumatism and, 137
  tomatoes for, 57
Insecticides, 4–7
Insects
  lavender and, 105
  mint and, 97, 98
  tomatoes and, 57
Insomnia, 144
  asparagus, warning against, 63
  lettuce for, 54

marjoram for, 86–97
radishes for, 62
Intestines, 129–31
  basil for, 95
  blueberries for, 68
  couch grass for, 107
  fennel for, 62
  tarragon for, 95
  worms in, 41, 44
Iron in strawberries, 65
Ivy, 107–9, 161

Jams, 189
  carrot, 224
  cider, 223
  elderberry, 223–24
  honey, 224
Jasmine paste, 226
Jaundice
  celandine for, 103–4
  parsley and chervil for, 84
Jesus Christ, 184
Juniper, 133

Kidneys, 131–34
  borage for, 116
  couch grass for, 107
Kidney stones, strawberries for, 65
Kipling, Rudyard, 171
Kohlrabi, 34

Labiate plants, 82
La Bruyère, Jean de, 167
La Rochefoucauld, François de, 242
Larrey, Dr., 130
Laurel (bay) leaf, 93–94
Laurent, Marie, 231–32
Lavender, 104–6, 165, 175
Laxatives
  asparagus as, 63
  blackberries as, 67
  chicory as, 59
  cucurbitaceous plants as, 82
  honey as, 189
  peaches as, 70
  plums as, 71
  rye as, 186
  violets as, 114
Leeks, 34, 44–45
Lemons, 126, 166, 173
Lettuce, 53–54, 143, 163
  au gratin, 217

Lettuce (*continued*)
  stuffed, 217
Leukhorrea
  blackberries for, 68
  roses for, 112
Levulose, 65–66
Lilies, 171
Lilies of the valley, 151
Linden, 142, 143
"Little cousin" (mallow soup), 200
Liver, 125–27
  artichokes for, 56
  asparagus for, 63
  cabbage for, 48, 49
  carrots for, 49
  celandine for, 103–4
  chicory for, 59
  cirrhosis of, 49, 190
  couch grass for, 107
  currants for, 67
  dandelions for, 60
  parsley and chervil for, 84
  spinach for, 58
  strawberries for, 65
  watercress for, 52
Liver fluke and watercress, 52
Louis XIV (king, France), 229
Louis XV (king, France), 92

Maceration, 124
Main dishes, recipes for, 203–10
Malle, M., 90
Mallow, 109–10, 133, 149, 156, 173
  soup, 200
Marigolds, 148
Marinated cucumbers, 219
Marinated pork roast, 209
Marjoram, 96–97, 125
  milk, 227
Meatless pot-au-feu, 202
Meats, 181–83
  additives in, 21–22, 161, 182
  for skin, 170
  see also names of indivdual meats
Melissa (herb), 128
Melons, 126
Mendicant, 180
Menstruation, 148, 149
  fennel for, 62–63
Mental illness, 119
Menthol, 99
Milk, 186–87

  cabbage with, 215
  marjoram, 227
  in skin treatment, 169
  sour-milk soup, 199
Mineral water, 127
Mint, 35, 97–100, 151, 173
  peas with, 218
  sauce, 210
Mistletoe, 158
Mixed herb sauce, 211–12
Montaigne, Michael Eyquem de, 33, 241
Montespan, Marquise de, 92
Morphine, 110
Mouth. *See* Teeth, mouth and gums
Mouthwash, mallow as, 110
Mulled wine, 227
Muscular aches, cabbage for, 48
Music and sex, 237
Mutton
  galimfrey, 204
  gasconnade, 209

Napoleon, 130, 147
Nasturtium, 35, 114–15, 175
National Association of Mayors (France), 28
National Conference for the Defense of Nature (France), 2–3
Natural foods, 22–30
Nero, 167
Nervous system, 142–44
  basil for, 94–95
  celery for, 51–52
  hawthorn for, 115
  lavender for, 106
  skin and disorders of, 163
Nettles, 34, 35, 100–2, 136, 236
  soup, 201–2
Nightmares
  cabbage for, 49
  lettuce for, 54
Nostradamus, 146

Oats, 186
Oleander leaf, 94
Olives and olive oil, 126, 130, 151, 165, 166
Olivier, Raymond, 194
Omelette, herb, 206–7
Onions, 34, 35, 43–46, 133
  cabbage with, 215

carbonade, 208
chicken with, 207–8
in the embers, 216
puréed, 215–16
soup, creamed, 197
tart, 207
velvet eggs, 207
wine, 44, 133
Orange blossoms
candied, 226
custard, 225
ratafia, 228
Oranges, 70, 126, 172
Oregano, 96–97
Organic foods, 22–30
Ortholan, Dr., 20
Osmosis, 124–25, 149, 162
Our Lady's Seal (plant), 165
Ovid, 101

Pansies, 168
Parsley, 34, 42, 44, 84–85, 141, 148, 165, 166, 168
Pasquini, Pierre, 9–10
Pastes, 226
Pasteur, Louis, 187
Peach blossoms, 80
Peaches, 70
Pears, 70
Peas, 34
with mint, 218
soup, 201
soup, tarragon, 201
Peppermint, 98
Perfumes, 175–76
Pesticides, 4–8, 17
Petronius, 101
Pfeiffer, Prof., 102
Phenol, 86
Picasso, Pablo, 240
Pigs and hogs, 182–83
Pimpernel, 104
sauce, 213
Pine bark, 152
Pius IX (pope), 157
Plague
cabbage for, 46
garlic and, 42
Vinegar of the Four Robbers for, 90, 138
Plums, 71
Poisoning, milk for, 187

Pollution, 1–12, 13–14, 122, 140, 184, 190
Pompadour, Marquise de, 167, 170
Poor man's sauce, 212
Poppaea, 167
Poppies, 110–11, 141, 143, 144
Pork
fat as skin treatment, 169
roast, marinated, 209
roast with herbs, 209
salmagundi, 210
Potatoes, 34, 171
Pot-au-feu, meatless, 202
Pot roast, Polish style, 206
Poultry, 183
stuffed with prunes, 205
Sunday night soup, 200
see also Chicken
Prunes, 71, 126
poultry stuffed with, 205
rabbit with, 204–5
Prussic acid, 94
Psoriasis, 162, 164
Pudding, coconut and vegetable, 218
Pumpkins, 170
Puréed onions, 215–16
Purgatives
rhubarb as, 64
violets as, 114
Purslane, 35
au gratin, 217
soup, 201

Queen Anne's lace (carrot), 50–51, 148
Queen Margot's potage, 199
Quince seeds, 165

Rabbit, 183
with prunes, 204–5
Rabelais, François, 101
Racine, Jean Baptiste, 139
Radishes, 34, 35, 60–62
soup, top, 202
Ragweed, 141
Raisiné, 180, 222–23
Raisins, 72
Raspberries, 65–66, 133
Ratafia
orange blossom, 228
rose, 228
Recipes, 194–229

Red cabbage
  with apples, 215
  salad, heated, 219
Renal colic, corn silk for, 118
Respiratory tract, 137–40
  infections of, radishes for, 61
  ivy for, 108
Rheumatism, 134–37
  celery for, 51
  corn silk for, 118
  lavender for, 175
  marjoram for, 97
  nettles for, 100–2
  onions for, 44
  parsley and chervil for, 84
  radishes for, 61
  raspberries for, 66
  rosemary for, 88–89
  roses for, 113
  spinach, warning against, 58
  strawberries for, 65
  thyme for, 87
  tomatoes for, 57
  watercress for, 53
Rhubarb, 64–65, 82
  blossom au gratin, 218
Rice, 131
Roast Pork with Herbs, 209
Ronsard, Pierre de, 230
Rosaceous plants, 82
Rosehip sauce, 212
Rosemary, 88–89
Roseola, 168
Roses, 111–13, 155, 171
  custard, 225
  honey, 227–28
  ratafia, 228
  vinegar, 165
Rum as shampoo, 174
Rutabagas, 63–64
Rye, 167, 186

Sade, Marquis de, 92
Sage, 89–91, 95, 125, 148
  sauce, 210–11
Salads
  American, and dip, 219–20
  dandelion with croutons, 218
  grapefruit dressing, 219
  greens, 53, 126
  red cabbage, heated, 219

Salmagundi, 210
Sauces, 210–13
Sausage meats, 182
Savory, 91–93, 166
  beans with, 216–17
Scallions, 44–45
Sciatica, 44
Scurvy
  cabbage for, 47
  onions for, 44
Seafood, 184
Sea holly, 101
Sexual activity, 235–37
Sexual problems, 144–49
Shallots, 44–45
Shellfish, 146
Shepherd's purse, 111
Shepherd's tea, 87
Sickness, 119–53
Skin, 162–66
  cucumbers for, 55–56
  facial, 166–71
  mallow for, 110
  nettles for, 102
  onions for, 44
  parsley for, 85
  strawberries and, 65, 66
  turnips for, 64
  watercress for, 52, 53
Snake bites, lavender for, 105
Soapwart, 175
Society of Environmental Protection
  (France), 17, 29
Sore throats
  cabbage juice for, 48–49
  nettles for, 102
  see also Throat
Sorrel soup, cold, 202–3
Soubiran, André, 162
Soubirous family, 25
Soupe au farci, 198–99
Soupe de vie, 197–98
Soups, 35–36
  recipes for, 196–203
Sour-milk soup, 199
Soviet Union, folk medicine in,
  37, 41
Speech defects, lavender for, 106
Spinach, 58, 125, 171
Spine, savory for, 93
Squash in the embers, 216

Starvation, 14
Stendhal, 158
Stomach, 127–29
    basil for, 95
    celandine for, 104
    spinach for, 58
    tarragon for, 95
Strawberries, 65–66, 132, 133
Stuffed breast of veal, 208
Stuffed cabbage, 213–14
    with chestnuts, 214
Stuffed lettuce, 217
Sugar, 188
Sulphur in wine, 11
Sunday night soup, 200
Sweets, 188–90

Tarragon, 95–96
    soup, 201
Tarts, onion, 207
Teas, 124, 192
Teeth, mouth and gums, 173
    apples for, 69
    blackberries for, 67
    horseradish for, 62
    infections of, blueberies for, 68
    mallow for, 109, 110, 173
    mint for toothache, 99
    thyme for, 88
Theresa of Avila (saint), 157
Throat
    infections of, blackberries for, 67
    infections of, currants for, 67
    violets for, 113–14
    see also Sore throat
Thyme, 85–88, 141
Thymol, 86
Tisanes, 124
Toffler, Alvin, 242
Tomatoes, 34, 35, 57, 126, 170
    in the embers, 216
Tonsillitis
    roses for, 112
    watercress for, 52
Toothache, mint for, 99
Tranquilizers
    mallow as, 109
    marjoram as, 96–97
    poppies as, 110
Truffles, 146–47

Tulips, 149
Turkey, 183
Turnips, 63–64, 125
Typhoid, onions for, 45–46

Ulcers, 128
United Nations, 14

Valence d'Agen, France, 28
Varicose veins, 152
Veal, stuffed breast of, 208
Vegetables, 34–73
    and coconut pudding, 218
    juice, 203
    recipes, 213–20
    see also names of individual
        vegetables
Vegetarianism, 181
Velvet eggs, 207
Villeneuve, Arnaud de, 191
Vinegar, 166
Vinegar of the Four Robbers, 90, 98, 138
Violets, 113–14, 129
    paste, 226
Vision, blueberries for, 68, 172
Vitamins
    A, in apricots, 70
    C, for colds, 138
    C, in currants, 66
    C, in oranges, 70
    C, in parsley and chervil, 84
    C, in watercress, 52
    C, in wheat sprouts, 186
    E, in grapes, 72
    E, in lettuce, 54
    in apricots, 70, 153
    in cucumbers, 55
    in onions, 43
    in strawberries, 65
    in vegetables, 36
Voltaire, 33, 145

Warts
    celandine for, 103
    dandelions for, 60
Water, 190
Watercress, 52–53, 126, 175
Water lilies, 149
Water pollution, 9–10, 184, 190

Water trefoils, 153
Wheat, 185–86
Wines, 190–91
   additives in, 11–12
   gentian, 226–27

hippocras, 229
mulled, 227

Yarrow, 116–17, 165
Yogurt, 187